MCQs in Clinical Nuclear Medicine

MCQs in Clinical Nuclear Medicine

D. A. Scullion
Senior Registrar, Department of Radiology,
St. Mary's Hospital, London, UK

G. Cook
Senior Registrar, Department of Nuclear Medicine,
Guy's Hospital, London, UK

R. Allan
Senior Registrar, Department of Radiology,
St. Mary's Hospital, London, UK

and

D. A. Cunningham
Director, Department of Radiology,
St. Mary's Hospital, London, UK

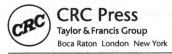

CRC Press
Taylor & Francis Group
Boca Raton London New York

CRC Press is an imprint of the
Taylor & Francis Group, an **informa** business

First published 1997 by Overseas Publishers Association

Published 2023 by CRC Press
Taylor & Francis Group
6000 Broken Sound Parkway NW, Suite 300
Boca Raton, FL 33487-2742

© 1997 by Taylor & Francis Group, LLC
CRC Press is an imprint of Taylor & Francis Group, an Informa business

No claim to original U.S. Government works

ISBN 13: 978-90-5702-109-1 (pbk)

Visit the Taylor & Francis Web site at
http://www.taylorandfrancis.com

and the CRC Press Web site at
http://www.crcpress.com

British Library Cataloguing in Publication Data

MCQ's in clinical nuclear medicine
   1. Nuclear medicine — Problems, exercises, etc.
   I. Scullion, D. A.
   616'.07575

Contents

Preface

This book has been written to fill the gap which we discovered whilst studying for the FRCR examination. There is a relative lack of up-to-date multiple choice revision questions written for nuclear medicine, even though these appear in the actual exam!

We found that the most useful MCQ books were those which provided explanations and/or lists which were difficult to extract from standard texts and we have tried to model this book along these lines; this is meant to be an exercise in nuclear medicine and not necessarily in passing MCQs. Hence the questions were not written strictly along examination guidelines and we have not tried to adhere to traditional examination interpretations of terms such as 'commonly', 'rarely', 'occasionally' etc.

We hope that future candidates find this useful in the run up to the FRCR. Although the DIR and MSc are not currently in MCQ format, we hope that candidates for these examinations might also find the 'question and answer' style useful for revision.

D. A. Scullion
G. Cook
R. Allan
D. A. Cunningham

Chapter 1
Bone scintigraphy

Malignancy

Q. 1.

a. In multiple myeloma the MDP bone scan is usually abnormal.

b. Increased ^{99m}Tc MDP uptake into metastatic deposits two months after chemotherapy indicates failure of response and progression of disease.

c. A solitary rib hot spot in a cancer patient usually represents benign disease.

d. A rib hot spot which is present over a year is likely to represent a simple healing fracture.

e. A solitary area of abnormal uptake in a patient with a known primary cancer with normal plain film appearances is likely to be benign.

A. 1.

a.   T   Bone scintigraphy is less sensitive than plain film radiography in detecting myeloma deposits as myeloma tends not to excite an osteoblastic response. It is still possible to see some areas of increased activity however and with modern cameras, resolution has improved to an extent where it is possible to discern cold lesions where bone has been replaced.

b.   F   The flare response, with increasing activity in the areas of metastases following chemotherapy, may persist for three months or more and indicates healing with successful treatment. Scans carried out before this time will therefore not be able to differentiate progressive disease from successful chemotherapy.

c.   F   About 40% of solitary rib lesions turn out to be metastatic (*Nucl Med Commun*, 1995; 16:834–837). Solitary rib lesions may also be due to minor trauma which may not even be recalled by the patient. In the context of breast carcinoma, lesions in the upper anterior ribs are often secondary to radiation necrosis.

d.   F   A simple traumatic fracture would be expected to show some resolution by this time. Metastases or pathological fractures from radiation necrosis would be expected to persist for longer. Metastatic rib lesions are often scattered and tend to grow along the bones with time rather than remaining focal.

e.   T   Bone scintigraphy is much more sensitive than plain film radiology in detecting metastases, often showing pathology many months before plain film changes. Surprisingly however less than 20% of bone scan lesions with negative plain radiology turn out to be malignant. (*Radiology*, 1990; 174:503–507)

Concerning radionuclide bone scanning in malignancy

Q. 2.

a. A malignant superscan requires more time to acquire the image.

b. It is possible to distinguish a malignant superscan from one of metabolic bone disease.

c. A superscan characteristically shows increased bone and renal uptake of MDP.

d. Uptake of MDP into malignant bone disease relies solely on osteoblastic activity.

e. It is not possible to distinguish benign from malignant vertebral collapse.

A. 2.

a.   F   A superscan is produced when there is diffusely increased uptake of MDP and hence a higher count rate
b.   T   and less time required to obtain the image. The uptake
into the bones is increased to such an extent that the
c.   F   bone to soft tissue ratio is increased with loss of
visualisation of the kidneys. On first inspection it
may appear normal because of the diffuse nature.
Diffuse malignancy and metabolic bone diseases such
as osteomalacia or hyperparathyroidism may cause
superscans. A malignant superscan may be distinguished from metabolic bone disease as there is usually some irregularity of uptake on close inspection,
especially in the peripheral skeleton.

d.   F   As with all causes of MDP accumulation blood flow to
the area in question is also an important determinant.

e.   T   Unless serial scans are taken when activity in association with osteoporotic collapse should fade with time
in most cases 6 months to 1 year.

Metastatic bone disease

Q. 3.

a. Radiotherapy will cause increased uptake of MDP locally.

b. A metastasis will characteristically show increased uptake on bone marrow scintigraphy.

c. A ^{99m}Tc nanocolloid bone marrow scan shows extension of bone marrow in polycythaemia rubra vera.

d. A ^{99m}Tc nanocolloid bone marrow scan shows extension of bone marrow in aplastic anaemia.

e. Peripheral extension of bone marrow which shows a patchy distribution almost always represents metastatic focal replacement.

A. 3.

a.   F   An endarteritis occurs with subsequent reduction of uptake of radiopharmaceutical. A sharp cut off to an area of reduced activity may give a clue.

b.   F   A bone marrow scan shows uptake of ^{99m}Tc nanocolloid into active marrow which usually occupies the axial skeleton and proximal long bones in an adult. Any process replacing marrow (e.g. metastases) will cause a photon deficient area.

c.   T   Extension of bone marrow is seen in this disease.

d.   T   This is one disease where there is mismatch between marrow function and cell production.

e.   F   Peripheral extension due to marrow hyperplasia from whatever cause can be very irregular giving the appearance of metastatic focal replacement.

Concerning bone scanning in trauma

Q. 4.

a. In NAI metaphyseal corner fractures are easily detectable with bone scintigraphy.

b. A bone scan in subradiological fractures of the scaphoid or neck of femur will be positive within a few hours of the trauma.

c. It is not possible to confidently resolve the separate carpal bones on bone scintigraphy.

d. It is common for a bone scan to be positive for a year following a scaphoid fracture.

e. Increased activity in association with osteoporotic vertebral fracture may take up to two years to resolve.

A. 4.

a.   F   Because of the proximity of the very active epiphyses in paediatric bone scans it may prove very difficult to resolve these lesions. Pin hole collimator views may be of help in this situation.

b.   F   24 hours may be required following a fracture for a sufficient osteoblastic reaction to be detectable on bone scintigraphy and scans performed within this time may be falsely negative. Even longer may be required in the elderly up to a number of days.

c.   T   The resolution of planar scans is not sufficient (about 7 mm fwhm). X-ray/bone scan coregistration is possible however, which enables exact localisation of hot spots.

d.   F   This would suggest that there is non union and/or avascular necrosis.

e.   T   This is a pathological fracture and may take some time for healing to occur. Nevertheless, a bone scan may be of use in approximately dating a fracture.

Concerning soft tissue uptake of MDP

Q. 5.

a. Appearance of the stomach on an MDP bone scan only occurs when free pertechnetate is present.

b. Radiotherapy may cause increased activity within the kidneys on an MDP bone scan.

c. Malignant pleural effusions accumulate MDP.

d. Arterial calcific atheroma does not take up MDP as it is not true bone.

e. Amyloid tissue may show uptake of MDP.

A. 5.

a. F   Faulty labelling of the radiopharmaceutical with free pertechnetate is the commonest cause for appearance of the stomach. The thyroid would also be seen. Severe hypercalcaemia may cause stomach uptake however.

b. F   Chemotherapy and hypercalcaemia may cause this appearance.

c. T   Malignant pleural effusions and ascites may show some MDP accumulation.

d. F   It is common to see the superficial femoral arteries on bone scans in patients with diffuse calcified atheromatous plaques.

e. T   Other causes of soft tissue accumulation of MDP include myocardial and splenic infarction, calcinosis of systemic sclerosis, breast, lung and other carcinomas, liver metastases, meningioma, neuroblastoma, myositis ossificans and rhabdomyolysis.

Concerning the use of SPECT in bone scintigraphy

Q. 6.

a. The spatial resolution of SPECT is better than that of planar bone scans.

b. Lumbar spine SPECT requires a high sensitivity collimator to overcome the low number of counts involved.

c. Lumbar spine SPECT can reliably differentiate facetal osteoarthrosis from a pedicular metastasis.

d. The facet joints are best appreciated on the sagittal views in tomography of the lumbar spine.

e. Lumbar spine SPECT is a good method of localising facet joint disease prior to joint injections.

A. 6.

a.   F   SPECT = about 12 mm compared to 7 mm with planar scans. Contrast resolution is improved.

b.   F   A high resolution collimator is used to preserve spatial resolution. A higher dose of ^{99m}Tc MDP e.g. 750 MBq versus 550 MBq for a planar scan, can be given to compensate for low count rates.

c.   F   The spatial resolution of SPECT is not adequate to differentiate activity in these two closely related structures with confidence.

d.   F   The axial and coronal views are usually better as the facet joints can be compared to those of the other side and at different levels.

e.   T   It is probably the method of choice.

Bone densitometry

Q. 7.

a. Osteoporosis is defined as a bone mineral density which is 2.5 standard deviations below the mean for 30 year olds.

b. The precision of dual X-ray absorptiometry is of the order of 5%.

c. Osteomalacia does not cause an abnormal reading on bone densitometry because it only involves osteoid.

d. Following HRT treatment initial scans should be performed at 6 monthly intervals to assess response.

e. The best predictor of bone mass in later life is bone mass in earlier life.

A. 7.

a.   T   This is the so called T score and is the WHO definition. Many clinicians use the Z score which relates bone density to a normal population of the patients own age.

b.   F   1%

c.   F   DEXA measures bone *mineral* density and so osteomalacia will cause low readings.

d.   F   Changes that are likely to take place in this short time are beyond the precision of the equipment to detect. Follow up of at least 2–3 years is more sensible.

e.   T   Following menopause, bone density is largely determined by peak bone mass. (*BMJ*, 1995; 310:1507–1510)

Infection

Q. 8.

a. Both infection and loosening of a hip prosthesis will show both increased vascularity and uptake on delayed images.

b. Increased activity in relation to a knee prosthesis one year after surgery nearly always signifies infection or loosening.

c. Cellulitis in a limb may cause increased uptake into bone on a bone scan.

d. Uptake of Gallium into a bone at the site of increased uptake on a bone scan nearly always signifies infection.

e. Bone scans are less sensitive in detecting osteomyelitis in neonates because of their small size.

A. 8.

a.   F   Only infection is usually associated with increased vascularity. Both will show increased uptake on delayed views. Focal uptake is typically seen at the tip of the prosthesis with loosening and more diffusely in infection although it is often difficult to differentiate between the two. White cell scanning or gallium scanning may then add further information in this situation. Newer cementless prostheses can remain diffusely "warm" indefinitely.

b.   F   This might be true for bone scans of hip prostheses but knees may take much longer to "settle in" following surgery. Increase in vascularity would be supportive of infection at this time however.

c.   T   Increased blood flow in the proximity of bones will cause some low grade uptake. It is usually possible to differentiate this from the markedly increased and focal uptake one would expect to see with acute osteomyelitis.

d.   F   Gallium has some bone seeking properties in its own right and has been used as a bone scanning agent in the past. Therefore any cause of increased metabolic activity will cause increased gallium uptake. If this is greater than that seen on the corresponding bone scan then infection is likely however.

e.   F   Neonates may produce false negative scans with acute osteomyelitis. This may in part be due to compromised local blood supply with subsequent reduced uptake of radiopharmaceutical.

Bone densitometry

Q. 9.

a. With accelerated bone loss, preferential loss occurs from trabecular bone as compared to cortical bone.

b. Bone density is measured following the injection of a bone seeking radioisotope.

c. A falsely low bone density reading may occur with coexistent vertebral osteoarthrosis.

d. A falsely low bone density reading may occur following vertebral laminectomy.

e. Single photon absorptiometry is the method of choice in measuring bone density.

A. 9.

a.   T   Bone density measurement are made in clinically significant areas such as the lumbar spine and femoral neck rather than the forearm where there is a greater proportion of cortical to trabecular bone.

b.   F   The most popular method of measuring bone density is by dual X-ray absorptiometry. Two beams of X-ray

c.   F   photons of different energy are transmitted through the patient. The amount of absorption is measured for each

d.   T   photon energy and the attenuation due to soft tissue can therefore be allowed for in quantifying that due to

e.   F   bone alone. Any cause of calcified tissue overlying the spine such as a calcified aorta or large osteophytes will therefore give a falsely high reading. Removal of the lamina of a vertebra will obviously cause less attenuation of the X-ray beam for that vertebra. Newer technology allows lateral views of the vertebral bodies to be taken allowing for such errors.

Metabolic bone disease

Q.10.

a. The "tie sign" is a recognised feature.

b. Reduced uptake of MDP into the diaphyses of long bones is a recognised feature.

c. Osteomalacia causes a reduction in uptake of MDP as there is a reduction of bone mass.

d. Aluminium osteomalacia in haemodialysis patients causes a metabolic superscan in advanced disease.

e. Treatment with bisphosphonates may cause a reduction in MDP uptake into the skeleton.

A.10.

a.   T   A metabolic bone scan will show increased uptake into the axial skeleton, long bones, calvaria and mandible

b.   F   with beading of the costochondral junctions. The tie sign describes the increased uptake seen in the sternum. Faint or absent images of the kidneys will result.

c.   F   As well as renal osteodystrophy and hyperparathyroidism, osteomalacia may show a metabolic bone scan. In this case it is due to an increase in immature osteoid. It may occasionally be differentiated, however, by areas of more focal uptake corresponding to Looser's zones.

d.   F   Aluminium induced osteomalacia is caused by deposition of aluminium at the calcification front and blocks mineralisation.

e.   T   Bisphosphonates reduce the rate of bone turnover but this is usually of too small a degree to be able to detect on bone scintigraphy.

Primary bone tumours

Q.11.

a. Vertebral haemangiomata may cause reduced or increased uptake of MDP into a vertebral body.

b. It is possible to differentiate benign from malignant bone tumours from the degree of uptake of MDP.

c. Bone scintigraphy is a good method for assessing the extent of involvement of a bone in osteogenic sarcoma.

d. Bone scintigraphy is a reliable method of detecting soft tissue metastases e.g. lung in osteogenic sarcoma.

e. Bone scintigraphy is a useful preliminary staging procedure in Ewings sarcoma.

A.11.

a.   T   Most commonly no abnormality is seen. Those with increased activity may be a subset that are the symptomatic variety as many are incidental findings on plain films. Vertebral haemangiomata may be difficult to detect when they exhibit reduced uptake.

b.   F

c.   F   The bone scan may overestimate the proximal extent of the lesion probably due to increased vascularity.

d.   F   MRI is probably the method of choice today. Although metastases from osteogenic sarcoma frequently take up MDP, this is not often enough to make it a reliable method of detection.

e.   T   Up to 10% of patients may have bone secondaries at presentation.

Increased uptake of MDP is seen in

Q.12.

a. bone island

b. osteopoikilosis

c. fibrous dysplasia

d. melorheostosis

e. eosinophilic granuloma

A.12.

a.   F

b.   F   Similar histology to a benign bone island.

c.   T   Reflecting that metabolic activity is increased.

d.   T

e.   T   About 1/3 may be negative, however and plain films may be required in addition.

(Radiology Review Manual)

Bone scintigraphy in infection

Q.13.

a. Labelled white cell scanning is the method of choice in diagnosing osteomyelitis in HIV patients.

b. ^{99m}Tc HMPAO labelled white cells are preferable to ^{111}InCl labelled cells in the detection of acute osteomyelitis of the extremities.

c. ^{99m}Tc labelled white cells are the method of choice in diagnosing infection in children.

d. It is not possible to carry out white cell scanning in severely neutropoenic patients.

e. White cell scanning is the method of choice in differentiating acute infarct from osteomyelitis in sickle cell disease.

A.13.

a.   F   Due to neutropoenia and the hazard of handling HIV infected blood for prolonged periods, white cell scanning is not routinely used in AIDS patients. Good alternatives in the skeleton which overcome these problems are Gallium and radiolabelled human immunoglobulin.

b.   T ^{99m}Tc has physical properties which give images of better resolution than those with ^{111}In and hence is preferable when imaging small parts.

c.   T ^{111}In results in a much higher radiation dose, especially to the spleen and so ^{99m}Tc is preferable as a label in this instance.

d.   F   Labelling and injection of donor white cells is possible in such patients.

e.   F   White cell labelling is characteristically very difficult in patients with sickle cell disease. This is because the ESR is very slow and makes separation of cells for labelling difficult. Donor cells, anti-granulocyte antibody labelling or human immunoglobulin can be considered as alternatives.

Bone scintigraphy in avascular necrosis

Q.14.

a. Septic arthritis of the hip in children may cause absent uptake of MDP into the femoral head.

b. Osteomyelitis and bone infarction are easily distinguishable in sickle cell disease.

c. Decreased MDP accumulation lasts for about 6 weeks following bone infarction in sickle cell disease.

d. In chronic Perthes disease bone scintigraphy has a sensitivity and specificity of over 90%.

e. Bone scintigraphy a few weeks following femoral neck fracture that is associated with higher uptake in the femoral neck indicates a favourable prognosis.

A.14.

a.   T   This is caused by ischaemia due to an increase in pressure within the joint capsule. If pressure is not high then normal uptake may occur and so a normal scan does not exclude septic arthritis. Marked increased uptake raises the suspicion of accompanying osteomyelitis.

b.   F   Infarction results in increased uptake as bone repair starts following the acute event and so both may cause

c.   F   similar appearances. After 1 week all sickle patients show increased uptake following infarction. Increased vascularity on a three phase scan may point towards infection but this sign is not always present. White cell scanning or gallium scanning may be of help in distinguishing.

d.   F   This is true for the early phase of the disease when there is reduced or absent uptake into the femoral head. As repair and revascularisation occur there is normal or increased uptake.

e.   T   Delayed imaging can be useful for prognostic reasons to identify those who will require a prosthesis. Lower levels of uptake are associated with those developing complications such as redisplacement, segmental collapse or pseudarthrosis.

(*Nucl Med Commun*, 1994; 15:341–360)

Bone scintigraphy in trauma

Q.15.

a. Tibial stress fractures are indistinguishable from shin splints on bone scintigraphy.

b. Compartmental syndromes are indistinguishable from shin splints on bone scintigraphy.

c. Reflex sympathetic dystrophy syndrome may show reduced uptake of MDP.

d. 50% of non pathological rib fractures heal by one year.

e. In talar coalition increased activity is usually seen at the site of coalition.

A.15.

a.   F   Shin splints are almost never associated with an increase in vascularity on a three phase scan. On the

b.   F   delayed images shin splints tend to show activity extending along the tibia where stress fractures tend to be more focal. A compartment syndrome characteristically shows reduced uptake with increased soft tissue uptake at the extremities of the lesion.

c.   T   The most common finding is of increased activity on all three phases of a bone scan in the bones of an affected limb. On occasion, however, reduced activity may be seen.

d.   F   80% (*J Nucl Med*, 1991; 32:2241–4)

e.   F   Activity is commonly found at the posterior subtalar joint or superior talus due to altered stresses and not at the fusion site. (*AJR*, 1982; 138:427–432)

Bone densitometry

Q.16.

a. Dual X-ray absorptiometry is preferable to dual photon absorptiometry.

b. The radiation dose from bone densitometry is similar to that of a conventional bone scan.

c. It is possible to use ultrasound to measure bone density in the hip.

d. Patients being treated for osteoporosis should have scans at monthly intervals to assess the effects of treatment.

e. It is possible to produce lateral images of the spine with newer DXA scanners.

A.16.

a. T The higher photon flux of X-rays compared to a radionuclide source improves spatial resolution, precision and scanning time.

b. F Bone densitometry = 0.003 mSv, bone scan = 4 mSv.

c. F This method has been used in the calcaneum but measurements correlate less well with bone density at sites that are at risk of fracture i.e. the spine and hip.

d. F This far too frequent to be able to measure a difference. Yearly intervals would be more appropriate.

e. T This allows morphometric measurement to be made in addition e.g. vertebral height.

Bone scintigraphy in malignant disease

Q.17.

a. Patients with a known primary cancer and a single skeletal hot spot have a roughly equal chance that it is benign or malignant.

b. Patients with a known primary cancer and a single vertebral hot spot are unlikely to have malignant disease.

c. A bone scan is a useful routine staging procedure for carcinoma of the prostate.

d. A bone scan is a useful routine staging procedure for all patients with carcinoma of the cervix.

e. A bone scan is a useful routine staging procedure for patients with stage III and IV carcinoma of the breast.

A.17.

a.   T   This varies with the site of the lesion but 55% of solitary scan abnormalities are due to neoplastic disease.

b.   F   This reduces if plain film radiology is negative. Solitary vertebral lesions have around an 80% chance of being malignant.

c.   T   Between 34 and 51% of patients at presentation have abnormal bone scans. 7% of T1 tumours and 65% of T4 tumours have abnormal scans.

d.   F   Less than 5% of patients overall have evidence of bone metastases. In stage 3 or 4 disease about 20% may have metastases, however.

e.   T   Between 9 and 62% of patients in different series have abnormal bone scans at presentation of stage 3 disease. (*Bone Scanning in Clinical Practice*, Ch. 5)

Bone scanning in Pagets disease

Q.18.

a. A bone scan may be normal in Pagets disease.

b. A bone scan is the method of choice to detect sarcomatous change in Pagetic bone.

c. Pagets very rarely only involves a single bone.

d. The appearance of new lesions in a patient with established Pagets disease is a common recognised finding.

e. A bone scan is the method of choice in assessing response to therapy in Pagets disease.

A.18.

a.   T   Burnt out disease may no longer excite an osteoblastic response.

b.   F   Both are hot on a bone scan and unless it is large a sarcoma may not be detected. It has been suggested that sarcomata take up MDP less avidly than Pagetic bone but this is probably not a reliable sign. Plain films and MRI are probably the methods of choice today.

c.   F   10–15% of Pagets disease is monostotic.

d.   F   It is very unusual to see new lesions in this disease and alternative causes should be suspected.

e.   F   Although it can be used, biochemical markers are more sensitive and cheaper.

(*Bone Scanning in Clinical Practice*, Ch. 8)

Concerning bone scanning in paediatric disease

Q.19.

a. It is possible to distinguish the fibula from the tibia with the resolution of a good quality paediatric bone scan.

b. Loss of a sharp demarcation of the growth plate from the metaphysis is a known normal variant of paediatric bone scans.

c. It is usually possible to confidently exclude septic arthritis of the hip with a normal bone scan.

d. It is possible to exclude all significant pathological conditions of the hip with a bone scan and plain films in children.

e. A full bladder is required for SPECT imaging of the hips to detect Perthes disease.

A.19.

a.   T   This is a good quality control. The radius and ulna should, similarly be easily separated.

b.   F   This is a sign of metastatic disease in the staging of neuroblastoma.

c.   F   A bone scan may look relatively normal in this condition as the increased pressure within the joint may compromise the blood supply causing a reduction rather than the expected increase in MDP accumulation.

d.   T

e.   F   A bladder full of radioactivity causes artefacts on SPECT reconstruction in the area of the hips. (*Bone Scanning in Clinical Practice*, Ch. 14)

Chapter 2
Lung Imaging

The following conditions are typically associated with matched ventilation/perfusion defects on lung scans

Q. 1.

a. IV drug abuse

b. Congenital rubella syndrome

c. Histoplasmosis

d. Thymolipoma

e. Haematogenous metastases.

A. 1.

a.   T   Perfusion defects seen in intravenous drug abuse are typically matched and are usually due to injection of contaminants such as talc, or to septic emboli. The injected material is almost always infected and corresponding ventilation defects occur, corresponding to CXR abnormalities. Matched defects due to inhalation of drugs such as purified cocaine have also been described and are thought to be due to a profound local vasoconstrictor effect.

b.   F   Congenital rubella is associated with peripheral pulmonary arterial stenoses which cause multiple perfusion defects.

c.   T   Histoplasmosis may be complicated by fibrosing mediastinitis with subsequent involvement of the pulmonary arteries. By the time the patient is symptomatic the airways are usually involved and ventilation is also affected. Tuberculosis may also give the same imaging findings.

d.   F   Thymolipomas are soft fleshy tumours that mould around but do not obstruct mediastinal structures.

e.   F   Haematogenous metastases are usually small and produce diffuse bilateral sub-segmental defects of perfusion with normal ventilation. They have a predominance for the lower lobes. A large metastasis, or confluent group of metastases may obstruct an airway in which case a corresponding defect of ventilation will be seen.

(*Semin Nucl Med*, 1993; 23)

The following conditions may cause perfusion defects on lung scanning

Q. 2.

a. SLE

b. TB

c. Sarcoidosis

d. Retrosternal goitre

e. Radiation pneumonitis

f. Anomalous pulmonary artery

g. Bronchial carcinoma

h. Congenital lobar emphysema

i. Haemangioendoliomatosis.

A. 2.

a.	T	The list of conditions causing perfusion defects on lung scanning is long and a comprehensive list is given in
b.	T	the reference below. Many of these causes are rare and in most cases are accompanied by matched defects of
c.	T	ventilation.
d.	T	
e.	T	
f.	T	
g.	T	
h.	T	
i.	T	

(*Gamuts in Nuclear Medicine*, pp. 183–187)

The common causes of perfusion defects include:

- Pulmonary embolus (acute or chronic).
- Pleural effusion.
- Chronic airways disease.
- Pneumonia.
- Bronchogenic carcinoma.

Concerning isotope scanning in carcinoma of the bronchus

Q. 3.

a. Tumours less than 2 cm in diameter would be expected to produce a perfusion defect.

b. Tumour size is the commonest cause of a false negative study.

c. Hepatic activity may obscure right lower lobe lesions.

d. Approximately 50% of tumours will take up Gallium.

e. Defects of ventilation tend to be more marked than defects of perfusion on V/Q scanning.

f. Multiple matched defects are a common finding.

g. Recent administration of cytotoxics will increase the detection rate with Gallium scanning.

h. A false negative scan is commoner with squamous carcinoma than adenocarcinoma.

i. Thallium-201 uptake into bronchogenic carcinoma is common.

A. 3.

a.   F   Tumours less than 2 cm do not usually cause a detectable perfusion defect on V/Q scans.

b.   T   Size is the commonest cause of a false negative study, but others include co-existant lung disease, tumour necrosis and right lower lobe lesions obscured by liver activity, only the latter two being relevant with Gallium scans.

c.   T   Uptake in the liver may obscure right lower lobe lesions; when seen on a V/Q scan, it usually implies vena caval obstruction or right- to left-shunting.

d.   F   Approximately 80–90% of bronchogenic carcinoma will take up Gallium. Uptake does not appear to depend on the histological type. The predictive value of a positive scan is 97%. Mediastinal uptake of Gallium in the presence of a primary lung carcinoma has a predictive value of approximately 90% for metastatic spread.

e.   F   Tumours produce a perfusion defect (sometimes with an irregular edge) proportional to their size. Usually the perfusion defect is matched, although occasionally it may be unmatched. Hilar lesions may cause complete lack of perfusion and ventilation to one lung.

f.   T   This is due to the high incidence of co-existent chronic airways disease in patients with primary lung tumours.

g.   F   Recent administration of cytotoxics will suppress the uptake of Gallium into tumours, either temporarily or permanently. However diffuse lung uptake of Gallium may occur following cytotoxics or radiotherapy and the scan should be interpreted with this in mind.

h.   T   These tumours are more likely to undergo necrosis.

i.   T   It is taken up into over 50% of lung carcinoma but has no place in routine diagnosis.

(*Clinical Nuclear Medicine*, Ch. 3 and 18)

Concerning pulmonary embolism

Q. 4.

a. A single perfusion defect separated from the pleural surface by a rim of normal perfusion is rarely due to embolus.

b. Normal perfusion excludes clinically significant PE.

c. Indeterminate scans correlate well with pulmonary angiography.

d. The combination of clinical impression and lung scan results is a better predictor of PE than either taken alone.

e. Patients with a low probability scan and no evidence of venous thrombosis may be safely left untreated.

f. The particle count of Tc-MAA may need to be increased in patients with pulmonary hypertension to achieve diagnostic images.

A. 4.

a.   T   This is the stripe sign. An embolus would be expected to involve the pleural surface and therefore when this sign is present it is very unlikely to be due to PE.

b.   T   They require no further investigation for pulmonary embolus and in the absence of lower extremity thrombus can be safely managed without anticoagulants.

c.   F   There is no such correlation with the findings at pulmonary angiography.

d.   T   Risk stratification is improved. However this only applies when the clinical probability of PE is in agreement with either a high probability or low probability scan. When the scan result and clinical findings are indeterminate, further investigations may be needed.

e.   T   The risk of clinically significant events is extremely small.

f.   F   This may be hazardous. It is generally accepted that the particle count be reduced in these patients. Lung function may deteriorate acutely in patients with pulmonary hypertension. Where a right to left shunt is the underlying cause, cerebral embolism of radiolabelled MAA may occur.

(Semin Nucl Med, 1991; 21)

To date the largest prospective trial to assess the role of V/Q scanning in pulmonary thromboembolism is the PIOPED study (see appendix A), which compared V/Q findings with results of pulmonary angiography. Large defects were defined as >75% of a lung segment; moderate defects 25–75% and small defects <25%. The conclusions have been summarised (Worsley DF, Alave, A. Comprehensive Analysis of the Results of the PIOPED Study *J Nucl Med*, 1995; 36:2380–2387): i.e. A normal V/Q scan excludes a clinically significant PE. V/Q scans are most useful when classified as representing very low, low or high probability of PE with concordant clinical likelihood of PE. Patients with intermediate probability scans or scans which are discordant with clinical likelihood of PE usually need further investigations to diagnose or exclude acute venous thromboembolism.

In the imaging of lung infection

Q. 5.

a. Gallium uptake is highly sensitive for Pneumocystis carinii pneumonia (PCP).

b. Localised uptake of Gallium is common in PCP.

c. Uptake of Indium-111 labelled white cells in the lungs is relatively non-specific for infection.

d. Unmatched defects of perfusion are the most common abnormality seen on V/Q scanning in patients with bacterial infection.

e. In patients with tuberculosis, only sites of active infection are Gallium avid.

A. 5.

a.   T   Gallium uptake occurs in 100% of cases, even when the CXR is normal, but the specificity is lower at 75%. There is good correlation between Gallium uptake and abundance of leucocytes in lavage fluid, thus it may provide useful information on the resolution of both infective and non-infective processes.

b.   F   Gallium uptake in PCP is usually diffuse. Localised uptake that is segmental implies bacterial infection.

c.   T   Lung uptake of Indium labelled white cells is relatively non-specific, unlike in other parts of the body and also occurs when the cells are damaged during labelling, in ARDS, heart failure, atelectasis and infarction. In one study fewer than 50% of scans with focal lung uptake of Indium labelled white cells correlated with infectious lesions. For this reason Gallium is preferred for the imaging of lung infection.

d.   F   Defects are usually matched in bacterial pneumonia. In addition, unmatched ventilation defects (reverse mismatch) or ventilation defects greater than the corresponding perfusion defects, are very suggestive of infection.

e.   T   Gallium may also be taken up into sites of active disease in other organs.

Q. 6. Diffuse intense lung uptake of Thallium-201 during stress myocardial imaging

a. Has prognostic significance.

b. Occurs in aortic valvular disease.

c. Is most commonly due to idiopathic cardiomyopathy.

d. Correlates well with LV end diastolic filling pressure.

e. May be seen in normal individuals.

A. 6.

a.   T   The combination of intense lung activity and myocardial perfusion defects suggests severe diffuse coronary artery disease or poor left ventricular function or a combination of the two. These patients have a poor prognosis.

b.   T

c.   F   Multi-vessel coronary artery disease is the commonest cause of diffuse lung uptake.

d.   T   Lung uptake is due to increased extraction of isotope into the pulmonary interstitium and occurs mainly when there is a rise in left atrial pressure. In heart failure this correlates well with LV end-diastolic filling pressure.

e.   F   Less than 5% of activity is seen in the lungs in normal individuals.

The causes of intense pulmonary uptake of Thallium during myocardial imaging are:

COMMON: Multivessel coronary artery disease.
Cardiac failure
Smoking
Pulmonary hypertension

UNCOMMON: Mitral valve disease
Aortic valve disease

RARE: Idiopathic cardiomyopathy
Asphyxia in infants.

(*Semin Nucl Med*, 1992; 22)

Total loss of perfusion to one lung occurs in

Q. 7.

a. Bullous emphysema.

b. Beckwith-Wiedemann syndrome.

c. Following a Blalock-Taussig shunt.

d. Pleural effusion.

e. Swyer-James syndrome.

A. 7.

a.   T   The defect will be matched in ventilation. Usually there is a small area of recognisable perfusion.

b.   F   Total loss of perfusion to one lung is not a recognised feature of Beckwith-Wiedemann syndrome.

c.   T   The shunt is between the subclavian artery and pulmonary artery on the side opposite the aortic arch and is used to correct Falllot's Tetralogy. The lung receiving the shunt is hypo-perfused and the perfusion scan may be used to assess shunt patency.

d.   T   Effusions may fill the whole hemithorax and cause a matched defect. The appearances of the scan will depend on whether the patient is imaged supine or erect.

e.   T   The Swyer-James (Macleod) syndrome is an obliterative bronchiolitis thought to occur as a result of childhood infection occurring before the lung has fully developed. It usually affects the whole lung but may be segmental or sub-segmental. There is a matched deficit. By contrast, ventilation is normal in atresia of the pulmonary artery.

The causes of unilateral loss of lung perfusion are:

- Massive pulmonary embolism (23%)
- Airways disease: bullous emphysema (23%)

                          carcinoma of the lung (23%)

                          foreign body obstruction.
- Congenital heart disease (15%)
- Arterial disease: Swyer-James syndrome (8%)

                          congenital pulmonary artery atresia

                          Blalock-Taussig shunt
- Absent lung: pneumonectomy (8%)

                          unilateral agenesis

(*Atlas of Clinical Nuclear Medicine*)

Regarding perfusion/ventilation scanning in the follow-up of confirmed pulmonary embolism

Q. 8.

a. Perfusion defects may clear at 24 hours.

b. A perfusion defect still present at three months is likely to persist indefinitely.

c. A persistent defect implies lung infarction.

d. Underlying heart failure may enhance the resolution of perfusion defects.

e. A repeat V/Q scan should be performed prior to stopping anticoagulation.

A. 8.

a.   T   Perfusion defects may clear completely by as early as 24 hours, but some defects may only partially resolve.

b.   T

c.   F   A persistent defect implies pulmonary arterial occlusion, but vascular supply to the abnormal area may be maintained by the bronchial circulation.

d.   F   Underlying heart failure may delay resolution of perfusion defects. This may also occur in chronic lung disease and in elderly patients.

e.   T   A repeat V/Q scan is useful to assess resolution and to act as a baseline should further possible pulmonary embolic events occur.

(*Atlas of Clinical Nuclear Medicine*)

The following are true

Q. 9.

a. A high probability V/Q scan has a positive predictive value of 90% for PE.

b. Perfusion/ventilation scanning gives a clinically useful diagnosis in approximately 75% of cases.

c. Most patients with PE confirmed on pulmonary angiography have a high probability V/Q scan.

d. A past history of PE increases the positive predictive value of a high probability scan.

e. Approximately 4% of normal or near normal scans will have documented PE.

A. 9.

a.   T   Overall high probability scans have predictive value for PE of approximately 90%. In the PIOPED study agreement between observers was greatest in the high probability and normal/near normal groups and reached 90%. In the intermediate groups agreement was lower at about 75%.

b.   F   Overall an indeterminate scan result was seen in approximately 50% of patients. Due to the risks of anticoagulation further investigation should be based on the clincal likelihood of pulmonary embolus.

c.   F   Only about 40% of patients with PE confirmed at angiography had a high probability scan.

d.   F   A past history of PE decreases the positive predictive value of a high probability scan as old pulmonary emboli may cause persistent defects.

e.   T   Approximately 4% (5 of 128 patients in the PIOPED study) with a normal or near normal V/Q scan will have documented PE.

(*J Nucl Med*, 1993; 34:1109–1118)

In the imaging of lung cancer

Q.10.

a. Thallium-201 is less specific than Gallium for differentiating inflammatory from neoplastic lesions.

b. Thallium-201 uptake into tumours is not influenced by recent radiotherapy.

c. Radiolabelled Somatostatin analogues have a higher affinity for non-small cell lung cancer than small cell lung cancer.

d. Negative uptake of Gallium in the mediastinum correlates well with the absence of mediastinal adenopathy at mediastinoscopy.

e. Increased lung uptake of Gallium in cytotoxic induced pneumonitis will occur even before CT abnormalities are evident.

A.10.

a.   F   Unlike Gallium, Thallium is not taken up into inflammatory lesions but accumulates avidly in neoplastic cells. It is therefore more specific in differentiating neoplastic from inflammatory lesions.

b.   T   Unlike Gallium, Thallium activity in tumours is not suppressed by steroids, cytotoxics or radiotherapy. However Gallium may be of use in demonstrating cytotoxic or radiation induced pneumonitis, even when other imaging modalities are normal (the time when treatment is most likely to be effective).

c.   F   Radiolabelled somatostatin analogues (Octreotide) are taken up by cells that express somatostatin receptors and are usually of neuroendocrine origin and derived from cells of the APUD (amine precursor uptake and decarboxylation) system. These receptors are expressed by a high percentage of small cell lung cancers and have also been found on a variety of other tumours. The role of these analogues in the detection of lung cancer is small. They have found greater use in other organ systems.

d.   T   Gallium is more sensitive than plain radiography for the detection of regional adenopathy. A negative Gallium scan of the mediastinum excludes adenopathy. Uptake of Gallium in the mediastinum in the presence of a known primary lung tumour has a sensitivity of almost 100% for mediastinal spread.

e.   T   Serial Gallium scans may be of value in monitoring the response to treatment.

(*Eur J Nucl Med*, 1994; 21:57–81)

Concerning Gallium-67 scanning in the evaluation of pulmonary sarcoidosis

Q.11.

a. The majority of patients will concentrate Gallium within the lungs.

b. Uptake of Gallium within the lungs and mediastinal nodes is sufficient to make a diagnosis of sarcoidosis.

c. A negative Gallium scan is highly predictive as a marker of disease inactivity.

d. Serial scans may be usefully employed to assess the response to treatment.

e. Diffuse lung uptake of Gallium is seen in approximately 5% of normal individuals.

A.11.

a.   T   The lower respiratory tract is involved in 90% of patients with sarcoid and the majority of these will exhibit lung uptake of Gallium in the active stage of the disease. Activity is diffuse and bilateral even when the lungs appear normal on conventional radiography. The exact mechanism of uptake is unknown but excess Gallium activity is to be found in alveolar macrophages.

b.   F   Co-existent lung and mediastinal uptake of Gallium is non-specific and seen in a variety of conditions such as infections, including TB; hypersensitivity pneumonitis, pneumoconioses and lymphoma; histological confirmation is usually required for diagnosis. However this pattern together with suggestive clincal findings and increased Gallium uptake in the salivary and lacrimal glands should point to a diagnosis of sarcoid.

c.   T   A positive scan correlates well with disease activity and has a sensitivity of approximately 97%. It is more useful in this respect than chest radiography, serum ACE levels and blood lymphocyte sub-set analysis. Likewise a negative scan in a patient with previous pulmonary sarcoidosis has a negative predictive value of approximately 87% for disease inactivity.

d.   T   Steroid therapy inhibits Gallium uptake in the lungs and the study may be used as a marker of response to treatment. Areas of residual activity may necessitate increasing the dose of steroids. A scan that becomes positive following successful therapy may indicate recurrent disease activity even when chest radiography and serum markers are still normal.

e.   F   In normal individuals lung uptake does not occur to any extent.

(*Semin Roentgenol*, 1985; 20:400–409)

Thoracic localisation of Thallium-201 may occur in

Q.12.

a. Mediastinal parathyroid adenoma.

b. Oesphageal carcinoma.

c. Sarcoidosis.

d. Hiatus hernia.

e. Sternotomy scar.

A.12.

a.   T   Thallium-201 may be used to localise an intrathoracic parathyroid adenoma prior to surgical removal.

b.   T   Uptake may occur in a variety of tumours including lymphoma, bronchogenic carcinoma and metastases. There is also abnormal uptake in many pathological conditions involving other organ systems.

c.   F   Sarcoidosis does not concentrate Thallium.

d.   T   Thallium is normally taken up by the stomach and a focus of increased activity in the thorax may be seen in hiatus hernia.

e.   T   The exact mechanism of Thallium uptake into scar tissue is unknown but it would seem to be related to the increased blood flow to tissues undergoing repair. It is important to recognise this phenomenon in patients undergoing myocardial stress testing following recent coronary artery surgery.

(*Semin Nucl Med*, 1988; 18:350–8)

Concerning Gallium scanning in patients with AIDS

Q.13.

a. Localised intense uptake of Gallium is most commonly due to Kaposi's sarcoma.

b. Kaposi's sarcoma lesions are Gallium avid.

c. A normal Gallium scan and CXR have a high predictive value for the absence of intrathoracic pathology.

d. Diffuse uptake of Gallium is seen in CMV pneumonia.

e. The pattern of lymph node uptake helps to distinguish reactive from malignant disease.

A.13.

a. F Localised intense uptake of Gallium is most likely to reflect bacterial pneumonia which is seen with increased frequency in AIDS and occurs in approximately 10–15% of patients. The diagnosis is very suggestive when the pattern of uptake is segmental or lobar.

b. F Kaposi's sarcoma does not take up Gallium. The combination of a negative Gallium scan and non-specific radiographic features such as reticular shadowing, nodules and pleural effusions in a patient with AIDS is suggestive of Kaposi's sarcoma.

c. T A normal Gallium scan and CXR suggests a source of infection or malignancy lies outside the thorax. However a few patients with advanced AIDS and proven lung infection at post mortem also have negative Gallium scans. This presumably reflects a severely abnormal or absent immune response.

d. T Diffuse lung uptake may be seen in other opportunistic infections such as PCP, CMV, cryptococcus and toxoplasmosis.

e. F There is no such distinction. Patients with HIV infection can show diffuse lymph node uptake of Gallium due to reactive changes. The pattern of lymph node uptake alone gives no useful clue as to the underlying pathological process.

(*Semin Nucl Med*, 1988; 18:273–286)

The following are true

Q.14.

a. Bronchoalveolar lavage (BAL) may cause perfusion defects on lung scanning.

b. Thymic uptake of Gallium may be a cause of a false positive scan in the assessment of the mediastinum in childhood lymphoma.

c. Healed tuberculosis may lead to a disproportionately large perfusion defect when compared to the CXR abnormality.

d. Unmatched defects of ventilation are common in acute bacterial pneumonia.

e. Increased lung permeability of aerosols is most commonly due to pulmonary fibrosis.

A.14.

a.   T   BAL usually causes matched defects on lung scanning, but the perfusion defect may occasionally be larger than the ventilation defect and cause diagnostic confusion. It is recommended that V/Q scanning not be performed within 24 hrs of BAL.

b.   T   Thymic uptake of Gallium is not uncommon in children, particularly when the gland is enlarged in co-existent viral infection. The characteristic sail shape should not be confused with uptake into mediastinal lymph nodes. Comparison with a CXR should aid differentiation between the two.

c.   T   In healed tuberculosis such as a healed Ghon focus, the perfusion defect is not uncommonly disproportionately large, even when the radiographic abnormality is small.

d.   F   Unmatched ventilation defects may be seen occasionally in bacterial pneumonia but in most cases perfusion is similarly affected.

e.   F   Changes in the integrity of the capillary or alveolar membrane will increase the washout of aerosols from the lung, although this effect is rarely of clinical significance. It is a non-specific finding and occurs in conditions such as ARDS, interstitial lung disease and sarcoid. It is most frequently observed in cigarette smokers.

The following are true

Q.15.

a. Scans taken in the lateral projection may be particularly useful in the diagnosis of pulmonary embolism in children.

b. The dependent lung is more efficiently ventilated than the uppermost areas of lung in children.

c. Ventilation of a lobe may be absent and then re-appear during the course of a ventilation scan in healthy children.

d. A perfusion scan performed 1 week following successful removal of an obstructing foreign body is likely to be normal.

e. In primary tuberculosis ventilation and perfusion defects are usually well matched.

A.15.

a.   F   In the lateral projection there is significant "shine-through" from the opposite lung. This projection is not routinely used.

b.   F   Unlike in adults, the uppermost areas of lung are optimally ventilated. The dependent lung is more efficiently perfused in both adults and children. This is thought to be due to a combination of relative diaphragmatic weakness and the smaller negative pleural pressure in children. This may be of practical importance in the treatment of children with unilateral lung disease.

c.   T   This is the "turn on — turn off" effect and is attributed to changes in ventilation occurring with change in posture. The result is an apparent ventilation/perfusion mismatch seen on some views but not on others.

d.   T   If a foreign body is not completely removed, by 6 weeks irreversible bronchiectasis supervenes and V/Q abnormalities may persist.

e.   T   In primary tuberculosis, ventilation and perfusion defects are usually well matched. Rarely, involvement of a pulmonary artery with TB may cause a striking V/Q mismatch.

The fissure sign occurs in

Q.16.

    a.   Sub-pulmonic effusion.

    b.   Cystic fibrosis.

    c.   Sarcoidosis.

    d.   Pulmonary embolism.

    e.   Emphysema.

A.16.

a.   T   The fissure sign is a defect seen on perfusion scanning
                 that corresponds to the shape and position of the

b.   T   interlobar fissures. It occurs in:

c.   F   –   Pleural effusion

d.   T   –   COAD

e.   T   –   Pulmonary microemboli

                   –   Cystic fibrosis

                   –   Thickening of the interlobar fissure

The mechanism for the sign is thought to be peripheral hypoperfusion due to a variety of pathologies such as compression, fibrosis and obliteration of small vessels. Pulmonary angiography in cases of the fissure sign do not produce the typical segmental defects seen in macroembolic disease, and suggests the presence of small peripheral microemboli or pulmonary hypertension.

(*AJR*, 1971; 111:492–500)

"Reverse" ventilation/perfusion mismatch occurs in

Q.17.

a. Pulmonary atelectasis.

b. Pulmonary embolism.

c. Alveolar proteinosis.

d. Bronchogenic carcinoma.

e. Pleural effusion.

A.17.

a. T The reversed mismatch is characterised by loss of ventilation but preserved perfusion. The loss of associated
b. F hypoxic vasoconstriction may be due to a variety of factors including associated pulmonary arterial pres-
c. F sure, respiratory alkalosis or local release of vasoactive mediators. Recognition of reverse mismatch excludes
d. T pulmonary embolism. The incidence of this phenomenon is approximately 10%. It has not been described
e. T in alveolar proteinosis. The causes are:

- Pulmonary atelectasis
- COAD
- Lung cancer
- Lung transplantation
- Metabolic alkalosis
- Pleural effusion
- Pneumonia
- Pulmonary hypertension.

(*Gamuts in Nuclear Medicine*, pp. 201)

Chapter 3
Renal Radionuclide Studies

In urinary tract obstruction

Q. 1.

a. A DMSA scan always estimates renal function more accurately than a DTPA scan.

b. Even if a kidney contributes less than 10% to the total GFR, it's function will usually improve if the obstruction is relieved.

c. Failure of the collecting systems to empty on standing confirms the presence of obstruction.

d. Lower urinary tract obstruction may be missed on a DTPA study.

e. Giving frusemide during a DTPA study results in a greater specificity for diagnosing PUJ obstruction than giving it at the start of the study.

A. 1.

a. F   DMSA may overestimate renal function in obstruction, as the tracer normally excreted by the kidney remains in the collecting systems and is counted, whereas in a DTPA study, function is assessed using renal uptake before excretion has occurred.

b. F   At this level of function, the kidney is irreversibly damaged and, unless removed, the patient is likely to develop hypertension.

c. F   If the collecting systems empty on standing, obstruction is excluded, but the converse is not true.

d. T   The tracer may have washed out into a grossly dilated lower urinary tract and if only the renal areas are measured, there may be a false negative result.

e. F   In this situation frusemide should be given 15 mins before the start of the study. This is because, with a flaccid dilated system, obstruction occurs with high urinary flow rates (accounting for the 'classical' symptoms in beer drinkers after a binge). These can be more reliably be achieved during the time course of the study if the frusemide is given beforehand; if it is given later, the renal pelvis may not become obstructed whilst the patient is being imaged and a false negative diagnosis of obstruction made.

Concerning radionuclide studies

Q. 2.

a. DMSA gives an accurate assessment of overall renal function in renal tubular acidosis.

b. DTPA studies can reliably exclude obstruction in a dehydrated patient.

c. A tissued injection can give a false positive result for obstruction.

d. An aortic aneurysm can be excluded if a dilated aorta is not seen on the blood flow renogram images.

e. Visualization of a ureter on a renogram is abnormal.

A. 2.

a.   F   DMSA is taken up by the proximal renal tubules. In some cases of renal tubular dysfunction there may be very poor uptake of DMSA with high background activity even with only mild renal impairment.

b.   F   In any situation where the GFR is low (dehydration, neonates, the elderly, chronic renal failure) there may be little or no response to frusemide, which may give a false positive diagnosis of obstruction, but if the kidneys empty, obstuction is excluded.

c.   T   Because there is only very slow delivery of the tracer to the kidneys, the T/A curves show a slow rising pattern which may be mistaken for obstruction.

d.   F   Apart from insufficient resolution, only the lumen is visualized.

e.   F   Persistent visualization of a ureter indicates a dilated ureter, but it is normal to see a ureter transiently, especially on a MAG 3 study.

Concerning radionuclide studies in acute renal failure

Q. 3.

a. ATN typically can be distinguished from other causes of acute renal failure.

b. On a DTPA study in pre-renal failure, there is impaired renal blood flow, poor uptake, delayed intrarenal transit and little or no excretion.

c. A rising T/A curve on a DTPA study confirms obstruction.

d. In ATN, a horizontal third phase to the T/A curve in a DTPA study indicates that recovery is occurring.

e. MAG 3 is the agent of choice.

A. 3.

a.   T   The typical appearances of ATN on a DTPA study are near normal blood flow, absent or poor uptake (equivalent to blood pool) and no excretion, in contrast to other causes where blood flow is reduced.

b.   F   This is the pattern seen in parenchymal disease e.g. glomerulonephritis. In pre-renal failure there is normal blood flow, good uptake, delayed intrarenal transit and no excretion.

c.   F   Because of filtration, prolonged intrarenal transit time and little or no excretion, tracer is retained within the kidney, the T/A curve continues to rise and there will be little or no response to frusemide (see 2b above).

d.   T   This indicates that the kidney is now capable of retaining some tracer in the parenchyma. As the kidney recovers further excretion will be seen and the T/A curves will begin to fall.

e.   T   There is better renal extraction (2.5 times higher than DTPA) giving a better tissue: background ratio and hence clearer images.

Concerning renograms and renal transplants

Q. 4.

a. On a DTPA scan, rejection can be distinguished from Cyclosporin A toxicity.

b. Arterial thrombosis can be distinguished from venous occlusion.

c. A high perfusion index means that there is a good blood supply to the transplant.

d. Arterial occlusion can be detected on a DTPA study even if an earlier one has shown ATN, from which the patient has not yet recovered.

e. Vesicoureteric reflux is the commonest cause of pelvi-ureteric dilatation.

f. A urinary leak can be excluded if it is not shown on the early images.

A. 4.

a.   F   Both cause reduced perfusion, reduced uptake and little or no excretion; usually histology is necessary to make the diagnosis.

b.   F   Both cause an avascular graft, which may be segmental or affect the whole kidney. If it is only segmental, then the cause is most likely arterial, but if the whole kidney is affected, end-stage rejection and hyperacute rejection must also be considered; none of these can be distinguished on the basis of the scan appearances alone.

c.   F   The perfusion index is the normalized ratio of the area under the T/A curves of the iliac artery: transplant given as a percentage. With normal flow to the kidney this will approach 100. High values mean that flow to the transplant is reduced. In practise a change in value is more important than an absolute one.

d.   T   Blood flow is preserved in ATN. One of the purposes of serial scans in ATN is to monitor blood flow in case another complication occurs (which would cause a visual change and an increase in the perfusion index.)

e.   T   This is commoner than obstruction; a renogram + frusemide is a good way of excluding obstruction.

f.   F   For a leak to be detected easily, there must be good renal function. If the leak is at the lower end of the ureter, it may be obscured by the bladder. Therefore, delayed views and post-micturition views may be necessary.

Summary of renogram appearances in transplant complications:

		Early Perfusion	Perfusion Index	Function	Urine output at 20 mins
ATN	initial	good	increased	moderate	0
	progression	good	decreased	increasing	+
Rejection	initial	moderate	increased	moderate	+
	progression	poor	increased	decreasing	+
Cy A toxicity	initial	moderate	increased	moderate	+
	progression	poor	increased	decreased	+

NB. Despite this summary, in the clinical situation one cannot be dogmatic since there is considerable overlap.

Concerning MAG 3

Q. 5.

a. A kit reconstituted first thing in the morning remains usable until the 99m-Tc decays.

b. MAG 3 has a smaller volume of distribution than DTPA.

c. Liver and biliary activity may be seen.

d. MAG 3 measures GFR more accurately than DTPA.

e. The radiation dose from a MAG 3 study is less than for a DTPA study.

A. 5.

a. F

b. T

c. T

d. F

e. F

MAG 3 is a ^{99m}Tc-labelled radionuclide which was developed to replace the 'gold standard' o-iodohippurate (OIH) which has the disadvantage of requiring labelling with iodine. OIH is excreted primarily by tubular excretion, so it provides a measure of tubular cell function and it can also be used to calculate effective renal plasma flow. It is 30–40% protein bound and 30–40% of intravascular activity is associated with RBC. Clearance is 75% by tubular excretion and 25% by glomerular filtration. MAG 3 is 75–80% protein-bound, so it has a very small volume of distribution (much smaller than for DTPA which is only 14% protein-bound), and only negligible amounts of the intravascular activity is associated with RBC. This means that more is presented to the kidney for excretion, so that although the plasma extraction of MAG 3 is only 50–65% of that of OIH, the urinary excretion, renogram curves and time to peak excretion are similar. Only 10% of MAG 3 is excreted by GFR. Due to the better isotope characteristics, and smaller volume of distribution (therefore lower background activity), the images produced by MAG 3 are superior to those of OIH.

MAG 3 is available in kit form. The US kit is stable for 6 hrs, but the European kit has a recommended stability of 1 hr following reconstitution and needs to be refrigerated to slow down the development of unstable 99m-Tc MAG 3 complexes. Most units attempt to 'batch' their MAG 3 studies, but to increase stability, the kit can be divided after reconstitution into aliquots of the doses required which are then frozen until needed.

Hepatobiliary activity may be seen occasionally, especially in patients with poor renal function. This is partly due to inevitable radiochemical impurities (approx. 3% of injected activity) and partly due to retention of 99m-Tc MAG 3 in the liver blood pool. The reason for gallbladder visualization is unclear, but if present may cause overestimation of the function of the right kidney.

DTPA is cleared almost entirely by glomerular filtration and its clearance correlates well with EDTA clearance until low levels of renal function are reached and in very young infants, due to the increasing statistical error on the measurements. As stated above, MAG 3 is both secreted and filtered; its clearance can be calculated, but it does not correlate precisely with GFR.

The whole body doses from DTPA and MAG 3 studies are similar, with MAG 3 giving a slightly greater dose to the renal tract and bladder.

(*Semin Nucl Med*, 1992; 22:61–73)

Comparing imaging techniques

Q. 6.

a. Renograms have a greater specificity for diagnosing obstruction than CT.

b. There is little point in doing a DMSA study if multicystic kidney (MCDK) is suspected, because of its known lack of function.

c. In diagnosing renal artery stenosis, ACE inhibitor renography is superior to Doppler US.

d. DMSA studies can reduce the need for invasive tests if ultrasound has demonstrated a solid mass.

e. Contrast CT is more sensitive in detecting acute pyelonephritis than DMSA.

f. In suspected MCDK, a MAG 3 study is unlikely to give any more information than a DMSA study.

A. 6.

a.   T   US, CT and MRI may show dilated systems with greater anatomical detail and may demonstrate the cause, but have much lower specificity, because they demonstrate a dilated system which does not necessarily equate with obstruction, especially when assessing an acute-on-chronic event.

b.   F   A unilateral multicystic kidney may be difficult to differentiate from hydronephrosis on US; a DMSA study will show no function in the case of multicystic kidney and a dilated system in hydronephrosis. If the changes are segmental, an IVU is necessary to distinguish between duplication with cystic dysplasia, multilocular cyst or segmental MCDK.

c.   T   Captopril renography is better both in the detection and prediction of therapeutic response. However, Doppler may be better for follow-up in patients in whom the renal arteries can be seen reliably, and will also detect co-existant abnormalities such as hydronephrosis.

d.   T   If the 'mass' is made up of functioning renal tissue, it is likely to be a normal variant such as a column of Bertin or a dromedary hump.

e.   F   DMSA is at least as sensitive at detecting both acute pyelonephritis and chronic damage.

(*Semin Nucl Med*, 1994; 24) *Seminars in Nuclear Medicine*, July 1994, vol. xxiv, No. 3.

f.   F   DMSA is the conventional nuclear medicine investigation in MCDK (see above) as it assesses renal function very accurately. However, not only can MAG 3 (i) assess renal function almost as accurately, but it can (ii) assess drainage of the abnormal kidney if the diagnosis is hydronephrosis instead of MCDK and (iii) assess the contralateral kidney. Up to one third of MCDKs have an abnormal contralateral kidney, typically vesico-ureteric reflux, congenital PUJ, renal hypoplasia and malrotation and MAG 3 is more likely to detect these than DMSA.

(*Clin Radiol*, 1994; 49:400–403)

In renal tract infections

Q. 7.

a. In acute pyelonephritis, there may be areas of decreased perfusion on the flow studies.

b. In a patient with a UTI a small smooth kidney is unlikely to be due to chronic pyelonephritis alone.

c. The overall sensitivity of DMSA is increased by SPECT.

d. A recognised feature of established scars is that they become more prominent with time.

e. Renal parenchymal involvement can be predicted from clinical and laboratory parameters.

f. Most acute parenchymal defects develop into cortical scars.

A. 7.

a.   T   Areas of decreased perfusion may be seen due to vascular compression. In gross infection which has spread into the peri-renal space, there may be reduced perfusion of the whole kidney. In this situation the kidney often appears enlarged.

b.   F   Chronic pyelonephritis is the most likely cause of a small smooth kidney but global loss of cortex can be caused by other conditions such as post-obstructive atrophy, renal artery stenosis and reflux nephropathy, all of which should be considered.

c.   F   SPECT is probably better at detecting scars, although the image acquisition time is longer so degradation of images by patient movement is much more likely as most of the patients scanned are paediatric, and the dose is higher.

d.   T   Renal scars become more prominent with time due to the growth of the surrounding tissues.

e.   F   In a recent study, laboratory indices, reflux demonstrated by cystography and the presence of P-fimbriated E. Coli together were no more accurate than symptoms alone in predicting parenchymal involvement, as shown by DMSA.

f.   F   Approximately 60% of acute parenchymal defects resolve.

Concerning vesico-ureteric reflux

Q. 8.

a. In patients who reflux, 20% reflux only during micturition.

b. Reflux seen on direct scintigraphic cystography correlates closely with the results of an MCUG.

c. Any reflux is a risk factor for pyelonephritis.

d. Renal scarring occurring after an episode of acute pyelonephritis is independent of continued reflux.

e. A recognised appearance on a DMSA scan of a kidney damaged by infection is a normal size kidney with reduced function.

f. Reflux occurring after the age of 3 yrs in patients with normal DMSA scans is probably irrelevant.

g. A 1 yr old with their first proven UTI and hydronephrosis on US should have a DMSA and an MCUG.

A. 8.

a.   T   80% reflux during filling and micturition, therefore virtually 100% of refluxers reflux during micturition.

b.   F   There is general correlation, but as reflux is an intermittent phenomenon, in many cases there is no correlation. There is not a good gold-standard test for reflux.

c.   F   The risk of pyelonephritis for those patients with reflux confined to the distal ureter is the same as for those who do not reflux.

d.   F   It is the combination of infection and continuing reflux that results in scarring as reflux without infection does not lead to scarring.

e.   T   The typical appearance is a scarred kidney; less common findings are a small kidney with no focal defects and a normal sized kidney with reduced function.

f.   T   Reflux occurring after the age of 3 yrs with no evidence of scarring is irrelevant and it is probably irrelevant after 1 yr.

g.   F   They should have a renogram (preferably MAG 3) to exclude obstruction and MCUG.

Concerning the imaging of renal transplants

Q. 9.

a. The peak blood flow to the kidney occurs 10 secs after the aorta.

b. Peak activity on a DTPA scan if GFR is normal occurs at 3–5 minutes.

c. Arteriovenous fistulae produce a characteristic appearance.

d. Uterine fibroids can be detected.

e. Haematoma and urinomas give identical appearances.

f. Uptake of Gallium is a sensitive index of rejection.

A. 9.

a. F With normal flow, peak kidney activity occurs 3–6 seconds after peak aortic activity, assuming a good bolus (time from initial appearance of aortic activity to peak aortic activity <3 secs). Note that this is not the same as the time/activity curve, which occurs over minutes.

b. T Time of first activity in the collecting systems is <5 mins.

c. T In this situation there is early visualisation of the IVC, which appears as a second stripe to the right of the aorta.

d. T These appear as abnormal tracer accumulation outside the transplant collecting system. Other causes include urine extravasation/urinoma, urine reflux into native ureter, wound dehiscence, menstruation and pregnancy.

e. F Both cause extrarenal photopoenic areas on early images, but a urinoma fills in with time. Other causes of extrarenal photopoenic defects are bowel (constant) and bladder (fills in if transplant functioning).

f. F Gallium is unreliable. Uptake is normally seen in the immediate post-operative period and in ATN, but may give a false-negative result in necrotic acutely rejecting kidneys, chronic rejection and if the patient is anticoagulated.

The following are the investigations of choice in the situations given

Q.10.

a. Creatinine clearance in the assessment of GFR.

b. The single-sample method of estimating GFR is most suitable for children.

c. Ultrasound in distinguishing congenital malformation and tumour.

d. A DTPA study in the evaluation of renal perfusion to native kidneys.

e. DTPA or DMSA scans in the evaluation of renal trauma.

A.10.

a.   F   The radionuclide of choice is 51-Cr-EDTA, which is virtually identical with inulin clearance and is therefore a true GFR marker, but is expensive. 99m-Tc DTPA has a clearance rate of 5% less than inulin (an acceptable error in clinical practice), is inexpensive, has low radiation dose and GFR can be estimated from serial blood samples taken during a diagnostic scan. Creatinine clearance has an error of 10–15% in estimating GFR, which may be greater in renal failure and is subject to more variations, such as diet.

b.   F   The methods of estimating GFR are based on compartmental models of the fluid spaces within the body and the rate at which DTPA passes though them (kinetic analysis). A single sample taken at 44 mins has been validated in adults as the relationship between fluid compartments is relatively constant. However, in children, the relationships between renal function, body compartments and body size change so rapidly that two samples are required; even so, the optimal time at which to draw the samples is debated.

c.   F   DMSA is the agent of choice as congenital malformations such as ectopic kidney will be easily seen as functioning renal tissue in an abnormal location and the majority of tumours are nonfunctional. Horseshoe kidneys are notoriously easy to miss on an ultrasound study, especially as the tissue overlying the spine is often a fibrous band. However, if suspected, anterior images should be performed.

d.   F   Nuclear medicine has a limited role in evaluating renal perfusion to native kidneys, although they are the procedure of choice in transplants, or in serial studies, or in the assessment of change after intervention, where repeated arteriography may be avoided.

e.   F   Nuclear medicine techniques can detect renal artery damage, renal contusion, segmental renal infarction, renal rupture and urinary extravasation, but if CT is readily available, they are not the procedure of choice. However, they do have a role in studying and follow-up of the functional results of renal trauma.

(*J Nucl Med*, 1991; 32(6))

Concerning paediatric studies

Q.11.

a. A normal child will have adult values of GFR by the age of 6 yrs.

b. All children with lower urinary tract symptoms require investigation.

c. Infants in whom an hydonephrosis has been detected antenatally should have a DTPA as soon as is practicable after birth.

d. If the antenatally-detected hydronephrosis has resolved on the ultrasound immediately after birth, no further follow-up is required.

e. Most children with antenatal hydronephrosis require surgery.

f. A normal DMSA in a child of 10 weeks reliably excludes any renal scars.

A.11.

a. T And 90% of adult values by 2 yrs. Under 1 month, measurements of GFR are unreliable and the infant kidney has an impaired response to frusemide.

b. F All children with proven UTIs require investigation and the younger the child, the more important this is. However, it has been shown that only 18–24% of children with urinary tract symptoms actually have a UTI, so to avoid unnecessary investigations and radiation, it is important to document a UTI before investigation.

c. F Renal ultrasound is the investigation of choice in the neonatal period, as it will confirm the diagnosis, assess whether it is unilateral or bilateral and look for associated anomalies such as dilated ureters, ureterocoele, enlarged bladder, small kidney or multicystic kidney. If urethral valve or vesicoureteric reflux are suspected, radiological micturating cystography should be performed next. Whatever the results, the radionuclide study should be delayed until the infant is 1 mth old, because of the low extraction rate, the low accuracy of GFR measurements and the impaired frusemide response. MAG 3 should be used where possible because of the higher extraction ratio.

d. F These children require a normal ultrasound scan at 3 mths to exclude continuing hydronephrosis as the scan after birth may be normal.

e. F Most children are unobstructed after birth, even though there was in utero obstruction. Serial DTPA studies suggest that the natural history of the condition is for the function to gradually improve, although severe unobstructed hydronephrosis may require a nephrostomy to decompress the affected side. Absolute indications for surgery are unequivocal obstruction (e.g. ureterocoele or posterior urethral valves), severe infection plus obstruction or PUJ with impaired renal function. Care must be taken when interpreting the serial studies in children under 2 yrs as an apparent improvement in renal function may be due to normal maturation of renal function.

f. F The poor tubular function of infancy results in poor uptake of isotope and high background activity; therefore a normal study performed earlier than 12 weeks will not exclude the presence of scars. However, it may be performed much earlier if it is important to distinguish between a non-functioning kidney and a poorly functioning one (e.g. in distinguishing between hydronephrosis and MCK, see above).

(*Eur J Nucl Med*, 1991; 18:41–66. Strongly recommended as a comprehensive review of Paediatric Nuclear Medicine)

Concerning renovascular hypertension

Q.12.

a. In children, a normal US and DMSA exclude the presence of renovascular disease.

b. Patients undergoing a renogram should be nil-by-mouth from midnight before the study.

c. Unilateral decrease in perfusion on a renogram confirms renal artery stenosis.

d. ACE inhibitors act on the efferent glomerular arteriole.

e. Captopril renography is more accurate in patients who are thought likely to have renal artery stenosis on clinical grounds.

A.12.

a.   F   In children, the younger the child and the more severe the hypertension, the more likely it is to be secondary; renal pathology is the cause in 90% over 1 yr. The commonest causes are scarring, PUJ obstruction and Wilm's tumour, which should be detected by US plus DMSA. Renovascular hypertension is usually due to fibromuscular hyperplasia +/− neurofibromatosis and usually requires angiography to evaluate it, although DTPA plus captopril may provide supportive evidence and post captopril DMSA studies may show focal defects due to branch stenoses.

b.   F   In normal patients there may be slight asymmetry of renal function (most centres take 50% +/− 5% as their normal range). The normal renogram is quite sensitive to the effects of hydration and posture; dehydration prolongs the parenchymal transit time, increases the radiation dose because little is cleared into the bladder, interferes with the diagnosis of obstruction and worsens any hypotensive reaction the patient might have to captopril.

c.   F   This is not the only cause of this appearance; the other diagnoses that should be considered include:−
- other vascular causes: renal vein thrombosis
  compression of hilar vessels
- parenchymal renal disease e.g. glomerulonephritis ATN
  collecting system obstruction
  peri-renal abscess and haematoma
  ptosis of kidney.

d.   T   In renal artery stenosis there is low pressure flow in the afferent glomerular arteriole. In order to maintain a pressure gradient across the glomerulus to maintain GFR, the efferent glomerular arterioles constrict, mediated by renin/angiotensin. When ACE inhibitors are given, this reflex is blocked, the efferent arterioles dilate and the GFR drops, resulting in worsening renal function and decreased uptake of DTPA.

e.   T   In a study of selected patients (hypertensive patients with known peripheral vascular disease, refractory hypertension not controlled by 2+ appropriate antihypertensives, and hypertensive patients with renal insufficiency without an obvious cause), there was a 50% prevalence of RAS and captopril renography had a 91% sensitivity and 87% specificity. However RAS is a rare cause of hypertension and if performed on all hypertensives, captopril renography has a 15–20% false-positive rate, (therefore a lower predictive value) which makes it less useful as a screening test.

(*Semin Nucl Med*, 1989; April 1989, vol. xix, No. 2)

In ACE-inhibition renography

Q.13.

a. Very tight stenoses (>90%) are more reliably detected than 60–70% ones.

b. With longstanding total occlusion of the renal artery, there can be no uptake in the affected kidney.

c. Branch arterial stenoses can be detected.

d. In a patient with a solitary kidney, ACE inhibitor renography may result in acute renal failure.

e. Frusemide is recommended at the start of the test to improve specificity.

f. In a MAG 3 study, a continually rising curve indicates a haemodynamically-significant stenosis.

A.13.

a. F In the context of renal artery stenosis, a positive test implies that the stenosis is haemodynamically significant, that renovascular hypertension (RVH) is present, and the lesion is likely to respond to angioplasty. However, if the stenosis is very tight, it may not be sufficiently compensated for (by the renin/angiotensin system) to produce scintigraphically-detectable changes after ACE inhibition; hence compensated 60–70% stenoses are the ones that are the most reliably detected.

b. F Uptake may be seen through collateral supply to the kidney; even in complete occlusion quite good uptake may be seen.

c. T In younger patients this is most likely due to fibromuscular dysplasia and may be associated with stenoses of the other major aortic branches or with neurofibromatosis.

d. T Especially if this has only one artery, and also if there is bilateral severe RAS.

e. T This clears any residual tracer from the renal pelvis, which makes counts obtained from the kidney more accurate. Hence it reduces the number of false positives, but does not affect the true positives. However, giving frusemide with an ACE inhibitor is dangerous due to the increased risk of a severe hypotensive reaction, and although it may improve specificity, this method is not generally accepted practice.

f. T The criteria for RAS on a MAG 3 study is a continually rising curve with increased cortical transit time and cortical retention at 20 minutes. A haemodynamically significant stenosis has at least 10% more 20 minute cortical activity on the post-captopril study than on the pre-captopril study.

On a DTPA study (glomerular agent) there is reduced early uptake at 2–4 mins, the graph flattens and the split kidney function changes. There may be non-visualization of the cortex. These measurements are less easily and reliably measured than the 20 minute cortical activity of MAG 3.

(*Radiological Clinics of North America*, 1993; 31(4))

Non-visualisation of a kidney on a DMSA scan may be due to

Q.14.

a. ATN

b. Tumour

c. Nephrotic syndrome

d. Crossed fused ectopia

e. Unilateral renal agenesis more commonly than postnephrectomy.

A.14.

a. F
b. T
c. T
d. T
e. F

The commonest causes of non-visualization of one kidney are multicystic kidney, neoplasm (this may replace the whole kidney, or displace it anteriorly so that it is not clearly seen if posterior images only are taken), obstructive uropathy, postnephrectomy and renal artery or vein occlusion.

Nephrotic syndrome may cause bilateral nonvisualization if renal function is severely impaired, but is also associated with renal vein thrombosis, which may be unilateral.

In infants, the whole abdomen is usually included in the field of view and crossed fused ectopia easily detected, but in larger patients, a kidney located outside the field of view may be apparently 'missing' unless pelvic views are done.

The causes of bilateral nonvisualization of the kidneys include acute and chronic renal failure, bilateral complete obstruction, bilateral renal artery or vein occlusion, bilateral cortical necrosis and glomerulonephritis.

(*Gamuts in Nuclear Medicine*, p. 343)

Concerning the visualization of the kidneys on a standard MDP bone scan

Q.15.

a. Non-visualization of a kidney usually means that it is non-functional.

b. If there is no retention of tracer within the collecting system, obstruction is excluded.

c. Most patients with retention of tracer on a supine image will have obstruction.

d. Retention of tracer in the collecting system in the upright position has a high predictive value for obstruction.

e. Frusemide given at the time of imaging increases the specificity for diagnosing obstruction.

A.15.

a.   T   MDP is excreted via the kidneys. Provided that the patient has two kidneys, if only one is seen on the bone scan it usually means that it is non-functional, since the other major cause of this appearance, i.e. superscan, affects both kidneys.

b.   T

c.   F   As for renography, erect images need to be obtained, as in a recent study, 75% of those who had suspected obstruction on a supine image washed out when erect images were taken.

d.   T

e.   F   It is not reliable.

(*J Nucl Med*, 1988; 29:1781–5). Haden, Katz and Konerding 'Detection of Obstructive Uropathy' by Bone Scintigraphy

Renal radionuclide imaging

Q.16.

a. Can distinguish between renal contusion and infarction.

b. Can detect radiation nephritis 3 wks after treatment.

c. Can detect central cysts more easily than peripheral ones.

d. A phantom kidney may be seen after nephrectomy.

e. A phantom kidney, if due to mesenteric vessels more commonly occurs on the right.

A.16.

a.   T   Serial scans are needed. Renal contusion shows decreased function in a portion of a kidney which returns with time, whereas in infarction, function does not return.

b.   T   This shows as generalized or focal reduction in activity as early as 2.5 wks and with 1.5 Gy. As in bone scans, there may be very straight borders to the involved area.

c.   F   Peripheral ones are easier to resolve; lesions as small as 1 cm can be detected.

d.   T   A phantom kidney is an apparent kidney seen when the patient is known to have no kidney on that side and are usually due to soft tissue masses/organs which are perfused on initial images but do not show selective accumulation of tracer.

e.   F   Usually the left.

The following are causes of the 'rim sign'. (central photopoenia surrounded by a rim of increased activity)

Q.17.

a. Multicystic kidney

b. Infarct

c. Haematoma

d. Renal vein thrombosis

e. Severe hydronephrosis

A.17.

a.   T

b.   F   This is an area of photopoenia only.

c.   T   Or this may just appear as a photopoenic defect.

d.   T

e.   T

Other causes include lymphocoele, and transplant rejection.

The following are causes of a flattened DTPA curve

Q.18.

a. Hypovolaemia

b. Hypoplastic kidney

c. Recent contrast angiogram

d. After extracorporeal shock wave lithotripsy

e. Severe cyclosporin toxicity.

A.18.

a. T Hypovolaemia and dehydration both cause reduced excretion.

b. T

c. T Intravascular contrast, especially in the doses likely to be used in an arteriogram, may precipitate renal failure, and hence reduced urine output, in susceptible patients.

d. T

e. T

Chapter 4
Endocrine Imaging

In the investigation of hyperthyroidism

Q. 1.

a. In Grave's disease, uptake of ^{99m}Tc is usually uniform.

b. If, after 2 years following ^{131}I treatment for Grave's disease the patient is still euthyroid, the incidence of subsequent development of hypothyroidism is negligible.

c. A normal isotope scan excludes Grave's disease.

d. Hypothyroidism following ^{131}I treatment of a solitary hyperfunctioning nodule is more common than in Grave's disease.

e. Low tracer uptake into the thyroid gland may occur in untreated hyperthyroidism.

A. 1.

a.   T   The gland is usually smoothly enlarged with diffuse increase uptake of tracer. Rarely Grave's disease may be superimposed upon a pre-existing nodular goitre and in this case uptake will be heterogeneous but overall uptake will be increased.

b.   F   It rises from 20% at two years to approximately 50–60% at 40 years. The risk of inducing thyroid malignancy from such therapy is considered to be negligible.

c.   F   Occasionally a patient may present with Grave's ophthalmopathy and be biochemically euthyroid. The scan may show normal uptake.

d.   F   It virtually never occurs. Suppressed normal thyroid tissue does not take up ^{131}I and is therefore protected. This is the treatment of choice for solitary nodules. However if a patient with a solitary toxic nodule is treated with radioiodine whilst taken antithyroid drugs the risk of subsequent hypothyroidism reaches 20% as the previously suppressed normal tissue will start to take up iodine as the TSH rises.

e.   T   This may occur in a number of conditions and is important to recognise as radioiodine will be an ineffective treatment. Such conditions include:
- Amiodarone therapy.
- Subacute thyroiditis.
- Post-partum thyroiditis.
- Recent heavy iodine load (i.e. contrast media).
- Excessive T4 administration.
- Ectopic thyroid tissue.

(*Radiological Clinics of North America*, 1993; 31(5))

117

The following are true

Q. 2.

a. About 25% of toxic nodules are palpable.

b. The scan appearances of Grave's disease may be confused with toxic multinodular goitre.

c. Thallium-201 may be used to demonstrate thyroid tissue in which uptake but not metabolic activity has been diminished.

d. Almost 10% of patients with Grave's disease will relapse following a prolonged course of antithyroid drugs.

e. Radioiodine therapy for thyrotoxicosis is contraindicated in pregnancy.

A. 2.

a.   F   Approximately 10% are palpable. Most impalpable nodules remain so even when their position is demonstrated on scanning.

b.   T   Grave's disease may coexist within a multinodular goitre and uptake is therefore heterogeneous. Rarely multiple toxic nodules may coalesce to produce diffuse uptake. Differentiation between the two is usually possibly on clinical grounds and confirming the presence of thyroid autoantibodies in Grave's disease.

c.   T   This is used in the demonstration of thyroid carcinoma and has the advantage over iodine in that patients do not need to stop their thyroid replacement therapy prior to scanning.

d.   F   The figure is nearer 50%. The cure rate for ^{131}I therapy approaches 100% but the risk of hypothyroidism is significant.

e.   T   It crosses the placenta and is excreted in breast milk. Antithyroid drugs are the treatment of choice but also cross the placenta and are excreted into breast milk. Care must be taken to avoid foetal hypothyroidism with it's increased risk of abortion and premature labour. Complete suppression of the gland in pregnancy is not necessarily desirable. Surgery is best performed in the second trimester.

(*Clinical Nuclear Medicine*, p. 198–231)

Concerning thyroid imaging in thyroiditis

Q. 3.

a. Thyroid uptake is usually diffusely decreased in acute (suppurative) thyroiditis.

b. Uptake in the early phase of subacute (de Quervain's) thyroiditis is usually increased.

c. Scan appearances in Hashimoto's thyroiditis may be difficult to distinguish from Grave's disease.

d. Radiation induced thyroiditis is commonly seen following external radiation therapy.

e. Radioiodine uptake in Reidel's thyroiditis is increased.

A. 3.

a.   F   This is a rare condition with 70% being caused by bacteria (staphylococcus or streptococcus). Uptake is usually normal although a focal abscess may show as a cold spot.

b.   F   This is a painful thyroiditis often following a viral URTI. Damage to the gland causes initial release of thyroid hormones with TSH suppression, clinical hyperthyroidism and decreased uptake. During recovery uptake returns to normal and then may be increased before returning to normal again. The course of the illness is 2–4 months. 1–2% of patients may remain hypothyroid.

c.   T   This is the commonest cause of adult hypothyroidism. There may be intermittent episodes of gland destruction over a period of years, eventually leading to hypothyroidism. Initially therefore TSH may be high and radioiodine uptake high, giving a scan appearance similar to Grave's disease. Eventually of course uptake is low despite high TSH as so much of the gland has been destroyed.

d.   F   It is uncommon and much more frequent with 131-I ablative therapy. The clinical symptoms are similar to those of subacute thyroiditis and the course is approximately 2–4 weeks. It inevitably results in hypothyroidism.

e.   F   The gland is slowly infiltrated with woody hard fibrous tissue and uptake may be very patchy and generally decreases. It is painless and up to 40% may progress to hypothyroidism.

(*Radiologic Clinics of North America*, September 1993; 31(5))

In the investigation of solitary thyroid nodules

Q. 4.

a. A single 'warm' nodule is likely to be an adenoma.

b. The risk of carcinoma in a hot nodule is 10%.

c. The risk of carcinoma in a cold nodule is at least 10%.

d. The risk of carcinoma in a dominant nodule within a multinoduar goitre is approximately 1%.

e. A history of childhood head and neck irradiation substantially increases the risk of malignant change in a solitary thyroid nodule.

A. 4.

a.   T   Nodules may be 'cold', 'warm' or 'hot' depending on the amount of uptake compared to the normal adjacent gland. The risk of carcinoma in a warm nodule is said to be in the region of 8–10%.

b.   F   Estimates vary but the overall incidence is small and is certainly considerably less than a solitary cold nodule.

c.   T   The figure varies from 10–25% in reported studies.

d.   F   Most would agree that the incidence approaches that seen with a solitary cold nodule in an otherwise normal gland. Whatever the case a dominant nodule should not be ignored and requires further investigation.

e.   T   The incidence rises to about 30–50%. The latent period may vary from a few years to well over 20 years. Fortunately this is now rare.

(*Radiologic Clinics of North America*, September 1993; 31(5))

The following are true

Q. 5.

a. The commonest site for ectopic thyroid tissue is the base of the tongue.

b. 123-I is superior than 99m-Tc in confirming the presence of a lingual thyroid gland.

c. Isotopes of iodine are superior than 99m-Tc for localising retrosternal thyroid tissue.

d. Absence of activity below the sternal notch excludes an intrathoracic goitre.

e. Ectopic thyroid tissue may be found in up to 50% of cases of neonatal hypothyroidism.

A. 5.

a.   T   Other sites include the upper neck along the line of thyroid descent, mediastinum and ovaries (struma ovarii).

b.   T   There is less artefact from salivary gland uptake in the neck and overall thyroid uptake is greater making target to background ratios better. 123-I is more expensive than 131-I or ^{99m}Tc however.

c.   T   There is greater gland uptake and better tissue to background ratio than with 99m-Tc. 123-I is usually used. There is less sternal absorption of 131-I due to it's higher keV but this is no longer used for diagnostic purposes for benign disease in this country because of its higher radiation dose due to beta rays.

d.   F   The goitre may be non-functioning.

e.   T   Absence of thyroid tissue occurs in 35%, and a smaller proportion are thought to be due to defects of hormone synthesis.

(*Clinical Nuclear Medicine*, Ch. 8)

Concerning malignancy of the thyroid gland

Q. 6.

a. The majority of tumours are of the follicular type.

b. Most tumours are well differentiated.

c. Most thyroid tumours are detected following demonstration of an area of increased uptake relative to normal thyroid on a 99m-Tc scan.

d. Anaplastic carcinoma never takes up 131-Iodine.

e. Screening of relatives is mandatory in anaplastic carcinoma.

A. 6.

a.   F   Papillary tumours make up 55–75% with follicular comprising 15–20%. The remainder are rare.

b.   T   By virtue of their follicular elements they may concentrate Iodine albeit less efficiently than normal thyroid follicles. The great majority synthesise thyroglobulin and this is a useful in follow-up, detection in the blood following thyroid ablation indicating recurrent disease. Rarely they synthesise thyroid hormones.

c.   F   Most are detected during the investigation of a cold nodule, either with FNA or following surgery.

d.   T   Rarely uptake is seen in medullary thyroid carcinoma but not sufficiently to make this a useful form of detection and treatment. Thyroid lymphoma does not take up radioiodine.

e.   F   There is no familial tendency in this tumour which occurs mainly in elderly patients. Screening of siblings is mandatory in medullary carcinoma when MEN II is suspected.

The following may cause a solitary cold nodule on thyroid scanning

Q. 7.

   a. Lymphoma

   b. Parathyroid adenoma

   c. Tuberculosis

   d. Wegener's granulomatosis

   e. Metastatic adenocarcinoma

A. 7.

a. T This is more often thought to be due to primary involvement rather than spread of disease elsewhere. It may present as a focal mass or as diffuse infiltration with patchy uptake on thyroid scanning. There does not appear to be a convincing association with auto-immune thyroid disease.

b. T Some 5% of parathyroid adenomas are thought to be clinically palpable and vary greatly in size. Tumours greater than 3 gms may be seen as a cold areas on thyroid scanning, depending on the exact site of the lesion in relation to the thyroid gland.

c. T Due to replacement of normal tissue.

d. F This has not been described.

e. T Careful postmortem examination of the gland in patients with malignancy suggests an incidence of approximately 10%. However most of these are small deposits and not clinically relevant. The common sites of origin are renal cell carcinoma and melanoma.

The commonest causes of a solitary thyroid nodule are:

1. Thyroid adenoma

2. Colloid cyst

3. Primary thyroid carcinoma

The following are true

Q. 8.

a. Patients with toxic multinodular goitre presenting with pressure symptoms should be treated with radio-iodine in the first instance.

b. Patients receiving I-131 therapy for thyrotoxicosis should take approximately 1 week off work following treatment.

c. The absolute level of thyroid hormones and TSH before treatment with radio-iodine is a useful predictor of the development of hypothyroidism in patients with Grave's disease.

d. A rise in the thyroglobulin level following complete ablation for thyroid carcinoma is indicative of recurrent malignant disease.

e. Uptake of radio-iodine into thyroid carcinoma metastases has prognostic significance.

A. 8.

a.   F   This may worsen symptoms acutely and surgery is the treatment of choice. However radio-iodine can be used to treat large non-toxic multinodular goitres with good results. Hypothyroidism is uncommon.

b.   T   They constitute a potential health hazard, albeit small. They should be advised of the statutory requirements concerning public travel, and should avoid prolonged contact with children and pregnant women for at least one week. Mothers should not breast feed till their milk contains only background activity. For practical purposes this usually means that they have to stop breast feeding indefinitely.

c.   F   They have no predictive value. The rate of onset of hypothyroidism is related to the absolute dose administered.

d.   T   Well differentiated tumours secrete thyroglobulin and serial estimations avoids the need to stop replacement therapy with it's unpleasant side effects. If the levels rise a formal I-131 scan should be performed off thyroxine treatment.

e.   T   Overall patients with local recurrence and metastases in lung or bone that take up radio-iodine have a significantly better prognosis than those patients with less well-differentiated tumours.

(*Eur J Nucl Med*, 1991; 18:984–991)

The following may aid in the differentiation of a benign from a malignant nodule on thyroid scanning

Q. 9.

a. Symmetrical opposing decreased uptake in the mid-portion of the gland.

b. A hot nodule on 99m-Tc scanning that is cold on I-131 scanning.

c. A cold nodule on 99m-Tc scanning that is hot on I-131 scanning.

d. A photopenic area in the centre of a functioning autonomous thyroid nodule.

e. A central core of functioning tissue surrounded by a rim of decreased uptake.

A. 9.

a.   T   This is the area of the greatest concentration of C cells and this appearance should raise the suspicion of medullary carcinoma.

b.   T   This discordant behaviour is almost always due to a thyroid adenoma, but rarely can be due to a primary carcinoma. The effect is thought to be due to disruption of the organification mechanism.

c.   T   This 'reverse discordance' occurs in thyroid adenoma, Hashimoto's thyroiditis and thyroglossal duct cysts. It does not occur with carcinoma. It is thought to be due to the presence of a small amount of functioning thyroid tissue with intact trapping and organification mechanisms. Over a period of time the target to background ration is better for I-131 than 99m-Tc.

d.   T   This is the 'owl's eye' sign. The cold area almost always represents an area of cystic degeneration within a solitary functioning thyroid nodule.

e.   T   This is the reverse of the above or 'fish eye' sign. It occur in a functioning adenoma with cystic degeneration at the periphery.

(*Gamuts in Nuclear Medicine*, p. 6–11)

Concerning imaging of the parathyroid glands

Q.10.

a. Approximately 50% of cases of primary hyperparathyroidism are due to a single functioning adenoma.

b. The sensitivity of parathyroid scintigraphy in the detection of adenomas within the gland approaches 75%.

c. In secondary hyperparathyroidism approximately 80% of hyperplastic glands will be visualised.

d. The majority of parathyroid carcinomas are functioning.

e. False positive scans may occur in the presence of coexisting thyroid disease.

A.10.

a.   F   It is almost 80%. Approximately 1–5% have 2 or more tumours and 10–15% have multiglandular hyperplasia. Most adenomas occur in relation to the lower poles of the thyroid gland.

b.   T   This is at least comparable to other imaging methods of localisation. The single factor best correlating with successful localisation is size.

c.   F   The figure is nearer 50%. The lower overall sensitivity is probably due to a combination of factors. The size of hyperplastic glands are often smaller than adenomas, counting statistics may make it difficult to identify all four glands and uptake may be reduced in patients with renal failure.

d.   T   About 90% of patients will develop evidence of hyperparathyroidism. It is rare but the scan appearances may be indistinguishable from an adenoma. Small metastatic deposits may go undetected by this method.

e.   T   This limits specificity. Most thyroid adenomas show increased uptake of Thallium and the scan may be uninterpretable in the presence of a multinodular goitre. Thallium is known to localise in many different conditions and rarely false positive scans have been described in sarcoid, lymphoma, thyroid carcinoma and metastasis.

(*Atlas of Clinical Nuclear Medicine*, p. 165–168)

Concerning scintigraphy of the adrenal gland

Q.11.

a. Asymmetrical uptake of 75-selenocholesterol may be seen in two thirds of normal subjects.

b. Bilateral symmetrical uptake of 75-selenocholesterol in the presence of glucocorticoid excess is usually due to adrenal hyperplasia.

c. Unilateral increased uptake following 75-selenocholesterol is most commonly due to a functioning adenoma.

d. Bilateral non-visualisation of the adrenals in the presence of endogenous glucocorticoid excess is most likely to be due to an adrenal carcinoma.

e. Unilateral non-visualisation excludes an adrenal carcinoma.

A. 11.

a.   T   This is due to the more posterior position of the right adrenal gland and the partial obscuration of the left gland by the upper pole of the left kidney. The true cause for the discrepancy should be apparent by comparing the anterior and posterior images.

b.   T   The likely cause is Cushing's Disease. Ectopic ACTH production may also cause adrenal hyperplasia.

c.   T   There is ACTH suppression by the tumour with non-visualisation of the contralateral normal gland.

d.   T   Concentration of selenocholesterol in adrenal carcinoma is poor per gram of tissue as is cortisol secretion. However the large size of these tumours results in enough excess steroid to produce hypercortisolism. Rarely a carcinoma may be differentiated enough to be visualised on scintigraphy. Overall the commonest causes of bilateral non-visualisation are technical and exogenous steroid therapy.

e.   F   The tumour may produce sex hormones or mineralocorticoids in which case the contralateral gland is not suppressed.

(*Semin Nucl Med*, 1978; 8:23–42)

The following tissues may show increased uptake of MIBG

Q.12.

a. Non-secreting paraganglionomas

b. Small (oat) cell bronchogenic carcinoma

c. Squamous carcinoma of the bladder

d. Medullary carcinoma of the thyroid

e. The heart

A.12.

a.   T   Rarely there may be intense uptake despite normal plasma and urinary catecholamine levels. This suggests uptake is related to the tissues ability to take up and store catecholamines and not to excessive endocrine secretory activity. This may explain uptake of MIBG into a variety of other normal and abnormal tissues.

b.   T   These tumours are derived from the neural crest and are related to carcinoid tumours. It is thought MIBG accumulates in neurosecretory granules within these tumours which are similar to those seen in the adrenal medulla and sympathetic neurones. This occurs even in the presence of normal catecholamine levels.

c.   F   This does not occur.

d.   T   Some 10% of these are part of the MEN IIa and IIb syndromes. Activity is also seen in metastases from this tumour and hence scanning may be useful in staging and follow up.

e.   T   The heart is richly innervated with sympathetic neurones. Peak uptake is at 2 hrs and is still seen at 24–48 hrs. Significant diffuse cardiac uptake lessens the likelihood of a phaeochromocytoma whereas absent uptake is said to increase the likelihood. Diminished activity is also seen with a variety of drugs and a drug history is essential. Normal activity of MIBG is also seen in the bladder, liver, gut, salivary glands and thyroid.

(*Gamuts in Nuclear Medicine*, p. 39)

In the scintigraphic assessment of adrenal hypertension

Q.13.

a. Pre-treatment with dexamethasone in patients with primary hyperaldosteronism significantly improves the diagnostic accuracy of selenocholesterol scanning.

b. Following dexamethasone suppression, a Conn's adenoma will usually be seen before day five.

c. Selenocholesterol scintigraphy can distinguish ACTH-dependent from ACTH-independent Cushing's syndrome.

d. False negative results may be seen during MIBG scanning in patients with phaeochromocytoma on steroid therapy.

e. Activity in the normal gland is usually suppressed in the presence of a unilateral phaeochromocytoma.

A.13.

a.   T   Dexamethasone suppresses ACTH dependent areas of the gland with better visualisation of an aldosterone secreting adenoma. The detection rate improves from approximately 75% to 90%.

b.   T   Normal adrenal tissue only "breaks through" after day 5. Bilateral hyperplasia may also be seen early in the examination. A Conn's tumour may be visible as early as 24 hrs.

c.   T   The pattern of uptake differs. Bilateral increased uptake occurs in hyperplasia and unilateral uptake with contralateral suppression occurs with a cortisol secreting adenoma.

d.   F   Exogenous steroid therapy has no effect on MIBG uptake into the adrenal glands.

e.   F   The normal gland is not infrequently seen. There is no suppression due to a contralateral catecholamine secreting tumour.

(*Semin Nucl Med*, 1989; 19:122–142)

The following are true concerning MIBG scanning

Q.14.

a. Focal bone marrow activity in the presence of a known neuroblastoma may be normal.

b. The sensitivity of MIBG scanning in the detection of neuroblastoma is approximately 90%.

c. MIBG scanning is more accurate than CT or MRI in the detection of primary adrenal phaeochromocytoma.

d. Increased adrenal uptake of MIBG in the MEN syndrome confirms the presence of a phaeochromocytoma.

e. MIBG scanning accurately reflects the extent of bony involvement in metastatic neuroblastoma.

A.14.

a. F   Increased activity is not seen in normal bone marrow and in this context implies metastatic spread.

b. T   Occasionally false negatives may occur due to very small lesions or liver deposits obscured by normal background liver activity. Overall MIBG scanning reflects disease distribution and specificity approaches 100%.

c. F   It is however superior in detecting the site of an extra-adrenal phaeochromocytoma and may prove useful in targeting anatomical imaging with CT or MRI.

d. F   The adrenals are more often hyperplastic in this condition which may cause bilateral diffuse increased uptake.

e. F   There is evidence to suggest that MIBG scanning alone will fail to detect or significantly underestimate the extent of bony involvement in a number of cases and that scanning with ^{99m}Tc-MDP is superior in this respect. However MIBG is better for soft tissue disease and it is recommended that both are employed in the staging and follow up of patients with advanced disease.

(*Semin Nucl Med*, 1993; 23:231–242)

Chapter 5
Gut and Infection Imaging

Concerning radionuclide scans and Meckel's Diverticulum

Q. 1.

a. Ectopic gastric mucosa in a Meckels diverticulum can be reliably distinguished from ectopic gastric mucosa elsewhere in the small intestine.

b. Cimetidine given before the scan blocks the secretion of pertechnetate from gastric mucosa.

c. Children are more likely to have a positive test than adults.

d. Diverticulitis is a common cause of a false positive result.

e. A false negative result may be obtained if there has been a recent barium study.

A. 1.

a. F   On a pertechnetate scan a key feature of ectopic gastric mucosa is that it has the same kinetics of appearance as normal gastric mucosa (activity appears immediately and is clearly visible by 30 minutes) this helps differentiate it from other inflammatory causes which accumulate pertechnetate more slowly. However, the exact location cannot be predicted precisely.

b. T   Cimetidine 'traps' the pertechnetate in the stomach and ectopic mucosa and increases the accuracy of the test by making activity more localized.

c. T   Meckels diverticula can be detected by radionuclide studies either by demonstrating ectopic gastric mucosa (pertechnetate) or by bleeding studies when actively bleeding. Those that contain ectopic gastric mucosa tend to present in childhood with bleeding (ectopic gastric mucosa is found in 30% overall, but in 60% of children).

d. F   Diverticulitis is a rare cause of a false positive Meckels scan as it is very rare in the typical (paediatric) population (see ans. c) and it does not give the same time course of activity; additional views may be helpful.

e. T   In general, it is inadvisable to perform a barium study immediately before any nuclear medicine technique which takes views of the abdomen as the barium shields any activity and may in, this situation, obscure activity in a Meckels.

Concerning the interpretation of gastrointestinal bleeding studies

Q. 2.

a. Hepatic haemangioma is a recognised cause of a false positive Tc-99m RBC study.

b. A rejecting transplanted kidney is a recognised cause of a false positive Tc-99m tin colloid study.

c. Anaemia is a cause of visualisation of the gallbladder in a labelled RBC study.

d. Diffuse colonic activity in a labelled RBC study invariably indicates colonic bleeding.

e. When reporting a study, it is not necessary to view the dynamic computer images as the 'hard copy' images provide all the information.

A. 2.

a.   T   Major blood vessels and vascular structures such as kidneys, liver and spleen are normally seen up to approximately 1 hour after injection. However, abnormal vascular structures will also show as increased activity. As in A1, the clue is the time course of appearance of activity and whether it moves or not.

b.   T   Tin colloid is cleared by the reticuloendothelial system at first pass, but also by rejecting kidneys. Hence it is normal to see liver, spleen and bone marrow, but activity outside these is abnormal (although free pertechnetate can cause bladder visualisation).

c.   T   This is presumably related to excess technetium complexes and insufficient RBC to bind to; multiple transfusions, i.v. contrast and renal failure are other causes.

d.   F   Any pancolitis (infective, inflammatory or radiation) will cause increased uptake to the entire colon.

e.   F   In a recent study, reviewing the cinematic display of the dynamic images was shown to improve the detection of a bleeding site by better visualisation/localisation and sensitivity in up to 38% of patients.

('*Nuclear Medicine in Clinical Diagnosis and Treatment*', Ed Murray and Ell, vol. 1; Ch. 5)

When investigating a patient with documented or suspected gastrointestinal bleeding

Q. 3.

a. Tin colloid studies are better at detecting bleeding sites proximal to the ligament of Treitz than distal to it.

b. Delayed images on a tin colloid scan may be of value in separating liver and spleen activity from bowel activity.

c. *In vitro* labelling of red blood cells (RBCs) gives fewer false positive tests than *in vivo* labelled studies.

d. Bleeding must be continuous to be detected on a labelled RBC study.

e. 51 Cr-chromate labelled RBC can detect bleeding down to 1–2 mls per day.

A. 3.

a. F   Liver activity on a tin colloid scan obscures and makes it difficult to interpret any activity in the right upper quadrant, where bowel proximal to the ligament of Treitz is situated.

b. F   Tin colloid is cleared rapidly from the blood, so active bleeding (approx. 2–3 mls per minute) must occur at the time of injection or very soon after. Therefore, delayed images do not localise activity accurately and are of limited value.

c. T   In *in vitro* labelling there is little free pertechnetate because it is washed off the cells before reinjection. However, this technique is time consuming (1–2 hours) and requires blood handling, so most centres opt for the quicker and more convenient *in vitro* method, where stannous is injected first and pertechnetate 20 minutes later and accept the tradeoff of activity due to free pertechnetate.

d. F   Labelled RBCs remain in the circulation and accumulate at the site of bleeding over a period of time. Therefore they can detect intermittent bleeding.

e. T   51 Cr-chromate labelled RBC studies are the most accurate ways of measuring blood loss, although this is not an imaging investigation. 59 Fe studies using whole body counting may also be useful as they can measure blood loss over weeks — months.

Concerning labelled RBC bleeding studies: early positive studies vs late positive studies

Q. 4.

a. In proven cases of GI bleeding, the scan is more likely to be positive in the first hour of imaging.

b. Patients with early positive scans usually have greater transfusional requirements.

c. Bleeding from the small bowel is usually more accurately located than bleeding from the colon.

d. The location of activity on the late studies is the most reliable indicator of the bleeding site.

e. Activity within the bowel is always due to gastrointestinal bleeding.

A. 4.

a. F >70% of labelled scans do not show a bleeding point at 1 hour.

b. F Even torrential arterial bleeding may be intermittent and this bears no relation to the timing of the study; it is important therefore to continue the study for long enough (6 hours at least).

c. F Small bowel bleeding is usually falsely located as occurring more distally than the actual bleeding point because of more rapid movement of RBC between serial images.

d. F The location of activity on the late studies is not a reliable indicator of the bleeding site as activity will have had time to pass down the intestine.

e. F Free pertechnetate may cause activity within the bowel especially on delayed images, but it is usually less intense than liver activity.

(*J Nucl Med*, 1991; 32:2249)

Concerning cholescintigraphy

Q. 5.

a. Failure to visualize the gallbladder by 4 hr with normal activity appearing in the bowel is highly suggestive of gallbladder disease.

b. Chronic cholecystitis can be distinguished from acalculous cholecystitis.

c. Giving cholecystokinin (CCK) before the isotope is more likely to demonstrate the gallbladder than giving morphine.

d. Common duct obstruction should be excluded if visualisation of bowel activity is delayed beyond 1 hour.

e. Gallbladder emphysema has a typical appearance.

f. The width of activity in an obstructed CBD on an IDA scan correlates closely with the diameter of the duct.

A. 5.

a. T Tc99m-labelled iminodiacetic acid compounds are cleared from the plasma and excreted by hepatic cells in a similar way to bile compounds. Normally the hepatic parenchyma is seen on the early images and gallbladder and bowel activity at 1 hour, but images should be obtained up to 4 hours if the gallbladder has not been seen earlier. Non-visualisation of the gallbladder at 1 hour with normal hepatic uptake and bowel activity is 99% specific for acute cholecystitis (cystic duct obstruction), whereas delayed visualisation of the gallbladder with respect to bowel activity has an overall 75% specificity for chronic cholecystitis.

b. F Both chronic and acalculous cholecystitis cause delayed · (i.e. 3 hrs +) visualisation of the gallbladder because its function is much reduced, but they cannot be distinguished. Rarer causes of delayed GB visualisation include hepatocellular disease, gallbladder carcinoma, pancreatitis, severe intercurrent disease and TPN.

c. T CCK given intravenously approximately 30 minutes before the test, causes the gallbladder to contract and empty of sludge and viscous bile so that tracer can then enter if the cystic duct is patent. Morphine acts by contracting the sphincter of Oddi, thus increasing the intraluminal pressure in the bile ducts. However, even with the increase in bile duct pressure, a sludge-filled gallbladder may not fill with tracer, hence CCK is more reliable.

d. T If the common duct is completely obstructed, hepatic +/ – CBD or gallbladder activity but no bowel activity is seen; increased renal uptake is also likely. Delayed bowel activity may be seen with a variety of other rarer conditions, such as severe hepatocellular disease, cholangitis, severe cholestasis, transplant rejection etc, but CBD obstruction is the commonest and should be excluded.

e. T The rim sign (a rim of activity in the gallbladder fossa) implies a very inflamed gallbladder wall and is due either to increased blood flow or exit of IDA through the inflamed wall. It occurs in severe, acute or chronic cholecystitis, emphysematous cholecystitis, gallbladder perforation and gangrenous cholecystitis, as well as adjacent hepatic inflammation.

f. F The width of IDA activity is directly related to the amount of radioactivity in the duct. The more intense the activity, the more scatter caused, which will result in apparent widening of the duct. This is a general principle of nuclear medicine and it is not possible to make direct measurements from the size of the area of activity on most nuclear medicine scans.

Concerning the post-operative evaluation after hepato-biliary surgery

Q. 6.

a. Cholescintigraphy has greater specificity than ultrasound at detecting bile duct obstruction.

b. Following cholecystectomy, an abnormal accumulation of HIDA outside the biliary tree is most likely due to a bile leak.

c. Ultrasound is more sensitive than cholescintigraphy at detecting bile leaks.

d. Cholescintigraphy can diagnose afferent loop obstruction after gastroenterostomy.

e. Ascites can be detected.

A. 6.

a.   T   Ultrasound is less specific than scintigraphy because it cannot detect early obstruction in undilated ducts, nor distinguish between non-obstructed and obstructed dilated ducts (e.g. ducts that were dilated pre-operatively may take time to decompress).

b.   T   The commonest cause of an abnormal extrahepatic collection of bile is a bile leak, but tracer accumulation in an obstructed bowel loop may mimic this appearance.

c.   F   Post operative fluid collections are often seen on ultrasound (seen in the gallbladder fossa in 53% after laparoscopic cholecystectomy) but appearances are not specific. Cholescintigraphy is more sensitive at detecting bile leaks because a collection has to contain bile to be detected, although it is not usually possible to locate the precise site.

d.   T   This provides a physiological study of afferent loop obstruction. Because the anatomy is preserved, the afferent loop fills from the common duct; normally tracer should then wash into the efferent loop and be seen in both loops by 1 hr post-injection. If the afferent loop is obstructed (e.g. at the anastamosis), tracer pools there (2 hours post-injection) with little or no activity in the efferent loop. This test may be useful in situations where it is difficult to get the afferent loop to fill using barium.

e.   T   If there is a bile leak into ascites, a gradual increase in activity over the whole peritoneal region is seen.

(*Semin Nucl Med*, July 1994; vol. xxiv, No. 3, 215–6)

In paediatric cholescintigraphy

Q. 7.

   a.   Phenobarbitone is used to maximise hepatic uptake of tracer.

   b.   Neonatal hepatitis can be distinguished from Rotor syndrome.

   c.   Choledocal cyst can be distinguished from a pancreatic cyst.

   d.   Cholescintigraphy is more accurate in diagnosing biliary atresia in children >3 mths than in neonates.

   e.   Dilated intraphepatic ducts are often seen in patients with biliary atresia.

A. 7.

a.   T   Phenobarbitone is a potent enzyme inducer and is used in paediatric studies to boost biliary excretion as in most conditions where IDA scanning is indicated (e.g. in the investigation of neonatal jaundice), hepatic function is likely to be impaired (see below).

b.   T   In **neonatal hepatitis** the defect is in hepatocyte function, so uptake is normal, but liver transit time is prolonged. Conversely, in **Rotor syndrome,** the defect is abnormal uptake and storage of bilirubin by the hepatocytes, so liver uptake is slow (cardiac blood pool, kidneys and urinary tract activity may be seen) with normal liver transit and excretion. However, the distinction is not always clear-cut, as severe hepatic dysfunction in neonatal hepatitis will result in reduced uptake.

c.   T   Both choledochal and pancreatic cysts may be detected as cystic structures near the biliary tree on ultrasound. Choledochal cysts communicate with the biliary system and can be seen on a HIDA scan, whereas pancreatic cysts do not.

d.   F   In **biliary atresia** the typical appearance is prompt hepatic uptake but no bowel activity because of bile duct atresia. These children develop progressive biliary cirrhosis and after 3 months liver function is so reduced that it is difficult to distinguish this condition from other causes of hepatocellular dysfunction.

e.   F   The intrahepatic ducts are also fibrotic so do not dilate.

Concerning GI transit studies

Q. 8.

a. It is easier to detect abnormalities of gastric emptying for solids than for liquids.

b. Diabetes mellitus is a common cause of delayed gastric emptying.

c. Hyperthyroidism is the commonest cause of rapid gastric emptying.

d. Scleroderma affects oesophageal transit through the whole oesophagus.

e. Achalsia has a specific appearance on a radionuclide oesophageal transit study.

A. 8.

a.   T   Gastric emptying of solids is a linear process, so the curve starts to fall immediately, whereas for liquids it is exponential, therefore the first part of the curve is nearly horizontal and minor disturbances are harder to appreciate.

b.   T   Diabetic gastroparesis is a common cause of delayed gastric emptying. Delayed gastric emptying can be due to true mechanical obstruction or secondary to functional abnormalities.

c.   F   Rapid gastric emptying is usually iatrogenic (i.e. post pyloroplasty or hemigastrectomy). Duodenal ulcer, gastrinoma (Zollinger-Ellison Syndrome) and hyperthyroidism are less frequent causes.

d.   F   Scleroderma affects smooth muscle only so only transit through the lower 2/3 of the oesophagus should be affected. 95% patients will have oesophageal involvement, but only 50% will be symptomatic, therefore 'silent' reflux may occur.

e.   F   Any oesophageal dysmotility disorder will show significant delay in clearance of the middle and distal oesophageal segments with stasis of >20% administered radioactivity at 2 minutes. These findings are not specific for achalsia, but can be used for follow up.

(*Semin Nucl Med*, April 1982, vol. xii, No. 2, 116–125, *Atlas of Nuclear Medicine*, Ed Nostrand and Baum, Lippincott 1988)

Concerning Paediatric Reflux studies ('milk studies')

Q. 9.

a. Reflux is more likely to be detected if the infant is placed prone.

b. The longer the test is carried out for, the more sensitive it becomes.

c. Labelled milk studies are better at detecting post-prandial reflux than 24 hour pH monitoring.

d. A normal study excludes significant lung aspiration.

e. Reflux detected by scintigraphy is more likely to be significant.

A. 9.

a.   F   Reflux is more likely to be detected with the infant placed supine on the camera.

b.   T   The longer the time period that counts can be obtained over, the more sensitive the test. The minimum acceptable duration is 30 mins.

c.   T   Gastric contents may be buffered by milk, so the pH may remain stable for long periods during the day and reflux not detected; labelled milk studies are independent of pH. They can also detect aspiration, but will miss nocturnal reflux.

d.   F   Significant lung aspiration has to occur during the limited period of the study, so a normal study does not exclude it.

e.   F   Reflux in infants is a different entity than in adults and occurs in healthy infants. The significance of reflux detected by either method depends on whether it is symptomatic.

(*Semin Nucl Med*, vol. xxv, No. 2, April 1995)

Concerning Gallium imaging of the abdomen

Q.10.

a. Uptake into surgical wounds is usually seen for approximately 1 week following surgery.

b. Even small liver abscesses can be localised accurately.

c. Most benign tumours give matched photopoenic areas on a combined gallium and colloid liver study.

d. Normal bowel activity is easy to distinguish from pathological abdominal uptake.

e. Diffuse abdominal uptake is seen in peritonitis.

A.10.

a.   T   Once injected, Gallium binds to lactoferrin and transferrin, which are found in the liver and spleen, the lacrimal and salivary glands (normal distribution) and in neutrophils (uptake into inflammatory foci). Uptake into surgical wounds does not necessarily imply wound infection and should be remembered when interpreting scans of post surgical patients.

b.   F   Small liver abscesses may be missed for two reasons: firstly they may be too small for the gamma camera to resolve and secondly Gallium uptake into the abscess may be the same as into the surrounding liver.

c.   T   To try and get round the problem encountered in (b), some centres perform a Gallium scan combined with a colloid liver scan and then compare or subtract the two sets of images. In general, matched 'cold' defects are caused by benign processes such as cysts and benign tumours, whereas lesions that take up Gallium but not colloid (i.e. unmatched) are aggressive — abscesses, primary liver tumours and metastases.

d.   F   Up to 15% of injected Gallium is excreted via the kidneys in the first 24 hrs; most of the rest is excreted via the colon after this time. Normal 'physiological' renal and gut uptake are two major causes of difficulty in interpreting abdominal Gallium studied. Bowel activity should fade with time and move between successive scans, but occasionally may be as intense as pathological activity. Giving the patient laxatives may help eliminate physiological bowel activity.

e.   T   Peritonitis, diffuse peritoneal metastases and generalised inflammatory bowel disease may all cause diffuse abdominal uptake.

Concerning the scintigraphic evaluation of liver transplants

Q.11.

a. Pre-operative hepatopulmonary syndrome can be diagnosed by MAA or colloid studies.

b. Nuclear medicine measurements of hepatic arterial and portal blood flow correlate with doppler measurements.

c. Nuclear medicine procedures are a first line investigation in vascular complications.

d. Bile leaks are more likely to occur in adults.

e. On a HIDA scan, delayed images need to be performed if biliary duct obstruction is suspected.

A. 11.

a. T Hepatopulmonary syndrome occurs when pulmonary arterial blood is shunted through the liver by collaterals and should be suspected in patients with severe liver disease, dyspnoea, a normal chest X-ray and resting PaO2 <60 mmHg. Shunting causes activity to be shunted to brain and kidneys; this can be quantitated by calculating the proportion of shunted activity. Response to treatment can be followed by sequential scans.

b. T There is good correlation between flow measurements obtained by scintigraphy and those made using doppler, except at very high and very low flow rates.

c. F Doppler US is the best immediate investigation and nuclear medicine is not used routinely.

d. F Bile leaks usually occur in the first few weeks after transplantation. They more likely to occur in children due to the small calibre of the recipient's bile duct and are detected by HIDA scintigraphy (see above).

e. T Biliary duct obstruction maybe due to stricture, mucocoele of the remnant cystic duct, obstruction by the T-tube, or stent blockage and usually needs delayed images to try to differentiate it from severely impaired hepatic dysfunction (slow extraction and slow excretion).

(*Semin Nucl Med*, vol. xxv, No. 1, January 1995, p. 36–47)

Concerning radionuclide imaging and organ transplantation

Q.12.

a. A normal rate of IDA excretion by a liver transplant predicts a normal biopsy.

b. In rejection, the portal contribution to hepatic blood flow falls to below 54%.

c. In primary non-function of liver transplants, homogeneous IDA uptake correlates with graft recovery.

d. MAG 3 can be used to diagnose vascular thrombosis of a pancreatic transplant.

e. Pancreatitis can be distinguished from rejection.

A.12.

a. T Prolonged IDA uptake and excretion is found in rejection, viral hepatitis and ascending cholangitis. With worsening liver function, it becomes harder to distinguish between rejection and obstruction, but a normal study excludes either and predicts a normal biopsy.

b. T A portal blood flow of <54%, as measured by sulphur colloid, combined with a heterogenous uptake of HIDA, is commonly seen with rejection.

c. T Primary graft non-function is the severest complication, which is associated with a high mortality and usually needs early regrafting. HIDA studies show delayed blood clearance and nonhomogenous hepatocellular uptake. However, if uptake is homogeneous, it correlates with graft recovery.

d. T DTPA and MAG 3 can be used to assess pancreatic transplant perfusion in exactly the same way as renal transplants. If the pancreatic graft and iliac vessels can be seen on the same early flow image, vascular occlusion or thrombosis can be excluded.

e. F Pancreatitis and graft rejection can be difficult to distinguish by any test. Findings include normal or increased flow, peripancreatic photopoenic areas, with increased labelled white cell or suphur colloid uptake.

(*The Radiological Clinics of North America*, vol. 33:3, May 1995, p. 473–492)

Concerning liver uptake of Tc 99m MDP

Q.13.

a. Focal uptake is more commonly seen in primary liver tumours than in metastases.

b. Focal uptake is more likely to be due to misinterpreted abdominal wall or rib uptake than to primary liver tumours.

c. Poor preparation of the radiopharmaceutical itself is a recognised cause of diffuse liver uptake of MDP.

d. i.v. contrast agents given after the MDP injection may cause diffuse liver uptake of MDP.

e. Diffuse liver uptake of MDP may be seen in hypercalcaemia.

A.13.

a.   F   The exact mechanism of MDP uptake into tumours is unclear; altered calcium and phosphate metabolism, increase permeablitiy and blood flow and necrosis are all implicated.

b.   T

c.   T   If faulty preparation causes microcolloids to form, these will be taken up by the liver RES.

d.   T   The exact mechanism of how contrast agents interfere is unclear. (*Clin Nucl Med*, 1978; 3:305–307)

e.   T   Diffuse liver uptake of MDP may be seen in hypercalcaemia, after high dose methotrexate, after repeated dextran injections and in acute hepatotoxicity — it is probably analogous to increased renal uptake of MDP which may be seen in similar situations.

(*Liver uptake of Tc-99m* — labelled phosphonate compounds — and updated Gamut, 1992, *Semin Nucl Med*, 1992, vol. xxii, No. 3 July: 202–205)

Concerning Indium-111 (In-111) white cell scans

Q.14.

a. The white cells must be autologous.

b. Lung activity is pathological between 1 and 4 hours after injection.

c. If a focus of increased uptake is seen on the early images, the 24 hour images do not need to be performed.

d. Indium-111 white cell scans are more useful in chronic PUO (>2 weeks) than acute PUO.

e. If the patient is on appropriate antibiotics, the white cell study is unlikely to be positive.

f. Active bleeding during the study is a recognised cause of a false positive result.

g. Diffuse lung uptake may be seen in acute respiratory distress syndrome.

A.14.

a. F   Usually autologous (from the patient) blood is used, but if the white blood cell count is very low, there may not be enough white cells to label efficiently and the existing cells are less likely to function, so donor (homologous) blood may be used.

b. T   Mild transient lung activity up to 4 hours is due to physiological margination within the lung vasculature. More marked uptake is usually due to damage to the WBC during labelling, which then become trapped by the lung macrophages. Persistent lung activity is abnormal.

c. F   An abscess will show as progressive accumulation of tracer over 24 hours; the early image will only rarely be negative but the delayed image is important for full evaluation of extent and location. Using this protocol, the reported sensitivity and specificity for detecting abdominal and pelvic abscesses is 90% and 95% respectively.

d. F   In-111 white cell scans are more useful in acute PUO where the cause is more likely to be sepsis. In chronic sepsis, the abscess may be walled off and separated from circulating WBC and in chronic PUO the cause is less likely to be sepsis (e.g. sarcoid, immunological disorders etc) and gallium is more useful.

e. F   Theoretically, effective antibiotic therapy may cause a false negative result, but this is open to debate and recent reports claim that they have no significant effect. Antibiotic treatment would certainly not preclude a study being performed. Immunosuppresion, including steroid and chemotherapy, may also potentially give false negative results.

f. T   Potential false positive results may be caused by bowel activity from swallowed purulent material from respiratory tract infection and sinus disease, active bleeding during the study or haematomas, tumour activity, or infarcted organ (within 2–3 days).

g. T   Pulmonary activity is recognised in pulmonary oedema, acute respiratory distress syndrome, after radiation treatment, leukaemia and metastases and infection.

Concerning ^{99m}Tc-HMPAO and 111-In labelled white cell scans

Q.15.

a. Diffuse bowel activity on a ^{99m}Tc-HMPAO study at 24 hrs indicates severe colitis.

b. On a ^{99m}Tc-HMPAO labelled white cell scan, the typical appearances of inflammatory bowel disease (IBD) is intense activity at 1 hr which fades with time.

c. Rectal disease can be distinguished from bladder activity on a ^{99m}Tc-HMPAO scan.

d. Activity is seen in the bowel in IBD because the labelled WBCs fix in the inflamed bowel wall.

e. An abscess that communicates with the bowel can be distinguished from one that does not.

f. The presence of a fistula may be inferred if there is no luminal activity on the delayed images when earlier images have demonstrated bowel activity.

A.15.

a.   F   A significant disadvantage of imaging with ^{99m}Tc-HMPAO is the presence of 'physiological' bowel activity which begins to appear after 1 hour and progressively increases with time. Hence early (approx. 1 and 3 hrs) are required and 24 hr images are not usually performed.

b.   F   The typical appearance of IBD on a ^{99m}Tc-HMPAO scan is activity which is present at 1 hr and increases by 3 hrs. Occasionally, the 1 hr scan may be negative, so sequential scanning is needed.

c.   T   Free ^{99m}Tc is excreted via the kidneys and may be seen as significant urinary tract uptake. Posterior views and lateral views are essential in assessing the rectum in patients with suspected rectal disease.

d.   F   In IBD the WBC migrate through the bowel lumen during the study (2–24 hrs and then pass down the colon; hence the typical appearance on an 111-In scan is positive uptake at 2–4 hrs with normal or much fainter uptake at 24 hours. Both early and late images are required so that affected bowel can be accurately located.

e.   T   As stated above, an abscess can be detected by a steadily increasing focus of activity. If an abscess communicates with the bowel, it's contents (i.e. labelled white cells) will enter the bowel and it's presence inferred on an 111-In labelled scan by diffuse greater bowel activity on the 24 hr images compared with the early images. It is important to recognise this clinical entity as the mortality is much higher than with non-communicating abscesses. ^{99m}Tc-HMPAO labelled scans are much less sensitive in this situation because of 24 hr physiological bowel activity.

f.   T

(*J Nucl Med*, 1994; 35:245–250)

The scintigraphic features which suggest fistulae are the simultaneous appearance of intestinal and extraintestinal activity and the absence of distal luminal activity in patients who do not have a colostomy or bowel obstruction to account for this lack of activity.

Concerning the imaging of the immunosuppressed patient

Q.16.

(see also Q13. Lungs)

a. 111-In labelled white cells are as sensitive as Gallium at detecting pneumocystis carinii pneumonia.

b. ^{99m}Tc DTPA clearance is more useful than Gallium scanning in the follow-up of PCP.

c. Gallium uptake into the colon is highly suspicious for acute colitis.

d. Kaposi's lesions take up 201-Tl.

e. Active MAI infection in HIV positive patients has a specific appearance on Gallium scans.

A.16.

a.   F   Gallium is more sensitive than labelled WBC scans at detecting PCP.

b.   T   In PCP infection the t1/2 of clearance of nebulised DTPA from the lungs is shortened, but rapidly returns to normal with successful treatment. This technique is more sensitive than Gallium at detecting and monitoring PCP infections. Faster clearances are also seen in other infections and smokers, but biphasic clearances are said to be found in PCP.

c.   F   It is extremely common to see colonic uptake of gallium.

d.   T   Kaposi's, lymphoma and infection (especially PCP) all take up Thallium; of these Kaposi's is the only one that does not also take up Gallium, so this could be used for diagnosis if necessary. (*'Nuclear Medicine in Clinical Diagnosis and Treatment'*, Ch. 20)

e.   F   In a recent study, no specific abnormality on a Gallium scan was found to indicate MAI infection. However, the combination of two or more of lymph node accumulation, paranasal sinus or colonic uptake and reduced bone marrow uptake made MAI likely (sensitivity 89%, specificity 70%). (*Clin Radiol*, 1995; 50, 483–488)

Concerning the imaging of infected prosthetic vascular grafts

Q.17.

a. CT is as sensitive and specific for the diagnosis of graft infection as labelled white cell scanning.

b. A negative ^{99m}Tc-HMPAO white cell scan at 3 hours excludes graft infection.

c. Infection occurring years after the operation is more difficult to diagnose.

d. Pseudoaneurysms may be diagnosed from the early images of a white cell scan.

e. Fewer false positive results are obtained if ^{99m}Tc-HMPAO labelled rather than 111-Indium labelled white cells are used.

A.17.

a.   F   In a recent study, ^{99m}Tc-HMPAO white cell scanning gave a sensitivity and specificity of 100% for graft infection, whereas CT had a higher false positive rate and sensitivity and specificity of 90% and 70–75% respectively.

b.   T   In the same study, no uninfected graft showed uptake at 3 hours; typically an infected graft showed faint uptake at 30 mins and intense uptake at 3 hours. However, some infected superficial extra-anatomic grafts were only weakly visible at 3 hours, so 24 hour images are required in this situation.

c.   F   The detection of infection by labelled white cell scans is not affected by the interval since surgery.

d.   T   If pseudoaneurysms are suspected, dynamic scanning is needed; they show up as foci of increased activity on the 5 min and 30 min images if using ^{99m}Tc-HMPAO-labelling.

e.   T   111-Indium labels platelets and erythrocytes, whereas ^{99m}Tc-HMPAO labels white cells more selectively, so intraprosthetic thrombosis, non-infected pseudoaneurysms and haematomas are more likely to accumulate 111-Indium labelled white cells. (*J Nucl Med*, 1994; 35:1303–1307)

Concerning imaging with ^{99m}Tc-human immunoglobulin (HIG)

Q.18.

a. Renal tract activity on the 3–4 hour image implies renal pathology.

b. Repeated studies are not usually possible, due to the risk of developing a host reaction.

c. The technique is better than Gallium at detecting infection in the thorax.

d. HIG studies are not usually useful in the detection of chronic osteomyelitis.

e. HIG studies are preferable to labelled white cell studies in HIV-positive patients.

A.18.

a.   F   50% of the activity is cleared by the kidneys in the first 24 hours; hence it is quite normal to see renal tract activity up to this time. There is also more blood pool activity than on labelled white cell scans.

b.   F   Sensitisation (the 'HAMA' reaction) is a risk with labelled monoclonal antibody studies, which are usually derived from mice, but this is very unlikely to occur with HIG. However, there are still the same risks as those associated with conventional pooled human immunoglobulin.

c.   F   Gallium is better at detecting infections in the chest, because Gallium imaging can be continued up to 96 hours, when blood pool activity will have subsided.

d.   T ^{99m}Tc-HIG is useful in acute osteomyelitis, but in chronic osteomyelitis it is less useful because, apart from the problem of variable blood pool activity, delayed (up to 48 hours) images cannot be performed.

e.   T   HIG is available as a kit and is given by a single intravenous injection, so it avoids the risks to nuclear medicine personnel and the risk of cross-contamination associated with cell-labelling.

Chapter 6
Cardiac Imaging

Myocardial Perfusion Scintigraphy

Q. 1.

a. The physical properties of Thallium-201 are such that its use is preferable to that of ^{99m}Tc labelled compounds in myocardial perfusion imaging.

b. The effective dose from a ^{201}Tl myocardial perfusion scan is one of the highest in diagnostic imaging and roughly equates to 3 barium enemas.

c. The uptake of ^{201}Tl relies solely on regional myocardial perfusion.

d. ^{201}Tl is a Na^+ analogue.

e. ^{201}Tl remains irreversibly fixed to the myocardium within a few minutes of injection.

A. 1.

a.   F

b.   T

c.   F

d.   F

e.   F

^{201}Tl has a relatively low energy (80 KeV) and relatively long half life (3 days). The long half life limits the activity that can be given to keep radiation doses at a reasonable level. Even so, the effective dose equivalent is about 20 mSv (Barium enema = 7 mSv, CT head scan = 4 mSv) which is higher than most other imaging procedures. The resultant low count rate and high attenuation due to the low photon energy is not optimal for imaging. The advantages of ^{201}Tl are that it is cheap and is better at detecting viable (hibernating) myocardium. This is myocardium that has no demonstrable blood flow or wall motion but retains some metabolic activity and on revascularisation may regain function. ^{201}Tl is a K$^+$ analogue and enters the myocyte via the Na/K pump in proportion to blood flow. Because uptake also relies on the Na/K pump, ^{201}Tl distribution also probably partly reflects metabolic activity and it may be for this reason that it is better able to detect hibernating myocardium than other agents. ^{201}Tl redistributes in the myocardium at rest and delayed images (3–4 hrs) reflect the distribution of myocardial perfusion at rest. By comparing stress and delayed rest images, areas of ischaemia can be determined.

The following may cause reduction in ^{201}Tl uptake to the myocardium

Q. 2.

a. Myocardial infarction.

b. Hibernating myocardium.

c. Cardiomyopathy.

d. Cardiac sarcoidosis.

e. Dobutamine.

A. 2.

a.   T   Both stress and delayed redistribution images will show a defect in uptake.

b.   T   Hibernating myocardium shows absent wall motion and reduced or absent blood flow but remains viable and on revascularisation may regain function. This may show the same appearance as an infarct on the stress and early redistribution images i.e. a fixed defect. It has been shown that by performing very delayed images (24 hrs) or by reinjecting ^{201}Tl, a number of fixed defects on the 3–4 hour images will show uptake of ^{201}Tl therefore differentiating hibernating myocardium from infarcted tissue. (*J Nucl Med*, 1994; 35(4) supplement)

c.   T   This presumably is in part due to the requirement for the Na/K pump to be functioning even if blood flow is
d.   T   normal.

e.   T   This is one of the pharmacological stressors that is used in patients that are unable to undertake conventional exercise and shows ischaemic areas by increasing myocardial oxygen demand.

Prognosis in coronary artery disease

Q. 3.

a. Increased uptake of ^{201}Tl into the lungs is a poor prognostic indicator during myocardial perfusion imaging.

b. Myocardial perfusion imaging may identify patients at increased risk of cardiac events following major vascular surgery.

c. Myocardial perfusion imaging has greater prognostic power than exercise ECG.

d. Myocardial perfusion imaging has less prognostic power than coronary arteriography.

e. In a patient with a strongly positive ECG but a normal myocardial perfusion scan, the perfusion scan is the most appropriate for defining prognosis.

A. 3.

a.   T   This is a reflection of high pulmonary capillary pressure at the time of injection and therefore relates to left ventricular function and hence prognosis. *J Nucl Med*, 1987; 28:1531–1535

b.   T

c.   T   This is probably due to a better assessment of the overall extent of ischaemia and better specificity. ST depression is a relatively late event during exercise compared to the changes in perfusion. *Am J Cardiol*, 1987; 59:270–277

d.   F   They are similar. *Circulation*, 1988; 77:745–758

e.   T   A 3 year follow up in 164 such patients showed a 0% cardiac event incidence. *Am J Cardiol*, 1993; 72:1201–1203

Concerning pharmacological stressor agents

Q. 4.

a. Dipyridamole reduces uptake of myocardial perfusion agents to myocardium.

b. Adenosine may be used as a cardiac stressor.

c. Caffeine intake should be restricted before an exercise myocardial perfusion scan.

d. Aminophylline may reverse chest pain caused by dipyridamole.

e. Dipyridamole is a potent coronary vasodilator.

A. 4.

a.   F

b.   T

c.   T

d.   T

e.   T

Dipyridamole is a potent coronary vasodilator and its effect is probably mediated by increasing local endogenous adenosine levels by reducing its degradation. Adenosine is an arteriolar vasodilator. Effects may also be partly mediated by intracellular cAMP and phosphodiesterase which may be negated by caffeine or aminophylline. Caffeine should therefore be restricted 24 hours prior to a dipyridamole perfusion scan and aminophylline may be used to reverse adverse effects if complications arise. Dipyridamole will increase coronary blood flow to vessels with a limited coronary reserve to a lesser extent than to normal vessels, without the induction of ischaemia and it is this differential that can be recognised on imaging. Ischaemia and chest pain is occasionally observed however, and this is thought to be due to a coronary steal phenomenon. (*Semin Nucl Med*, 1991; 21(3))

^{99m}Tc labelled myocardial perfusion agents

Q. 5.

a. Stress and redistribution images of ^{99m}Tc SestaMIBI accurately identify ischaemic myocardium.

b. ^{99m}Tc SestaMIBI is more suited to SPECT scanning than ^{201}Tl.

c. A fatty meal is required following sestaMIBI injection.

d. ^{99m}Tc SestaMIBI stress and rest myocardial perfusion scans cannot be performed on the same day due to the long residence time of this agent in the myocardium.

e. ^{99m}Tc SestaMIBI imaging should be performed as soon as possible following injection.

A. 5.

a.	F	^{99m}Tc SestaMIBI is a monovalent cation which is taken up in the myocardium in proportion to blood flow.
b.	T	There is no significant redistribution and so rest studies have to be performed following a second injection.
c.	T	This can either be performed on separate days after decay of the ^{99m}Tc, or more conveniently, on the same
d.	F	day but with a 3x larger dose on the second injection to "flood out" activity from the first injection. Because of
e.	F	the favourable physical characteristics of ^{99m}Tc it is more suited for SPECT scanning than ^{201}Tl. A chocolate bar or glass of milk is used to help clear hepatic and biliary activity which may interfere with imaging. An interval of at least 20 minutes is left following injection to allow some background activity to clear.

Equilibrium gated blood pool imaging

Q. 6.

a. ^{99m}Tc DTPA is preferable to labelled red blood cells in gated ventrigulography as radiopharmaceutical preparation is easier.

b. Red cells may be labelled with ^{99m}Tc *in vivo*.

c. Concurrent ECG recording is only necessary if there is risk of arrhythmia.

d. It is possible to assess regional wall motion abnormalities of the left ventricle.

e. Background subtraction is not usually required in measuring LV ejection fractions as activity within the adjacent lung is negligible.

A. 6.

a.   F   Any substance that remains within the blood pool may be used. DTPA may be used for first pass analysis but due to glomerular filtration blood clearance is too rapid for blood pool imaging.

b.   T   Red cells may be labelled *in vivo*, *in vitro* or by the modified *in vitro* method. The *in vitro* technique gives more efficient labelling but the *in vivo* technique is more convenient and less time consuming and is widely practised. Stannous ion is injected IV to prime the red cells 20 minutes before injection of ^{99m}Tc which then labels the red cells. 90% labelling efficiency is usually achieved.

c.   F   The scan cannot be "gated" without an ECG. Each cardiac cycle (R wave to R wave) is divided into a number of frames (e.g. 16) and counts are added to each frame in successive heart beats corresponding to the phase of the cardiac cycle. This allows a large number of counts to be gained for better image quality and statistical accuracy to give a cardiac cycle which is typically the summed information from 300 heart beats.

d.   T   By observing the changes in the shape of the LV cavity (blood pool) over a cardiac cycle which can be presented in cine mode, regional wall motion can be indirectly assessed. By producing functional images corresponding to amplitude and phase of motion, abnormalities can be more easily assessed. An infarcted area would cause an region of reduced amplitude and an LV aneurysm would show motion 180° out of phase with the rest of the LV (paradoxical movement).

e.   F   Background counts account for 30–60% of counts within an image. LV ejection fraction is calculated by

$$\frac{(ED - BG) - (ES - BG)}{ED - BG} = \frac{ED - ES}{ED - BG}$$

ED = end diastolic counts   ES = end systolic counts   BG = background counts
Counts over a region are assumed to be proportional to volume.

Equilibrium gated blood pool imaging

Q. 7.

a. Patients with coronary artery disease typically show an increase in LV ejection fraction of only 5–10% on exercise.

b. Regional wall motion abnormalities are more specific for coronary artery disease than changes in ejection fraction with exercise.

c. Patients receiving chemotherapy should be suspected of having cardiotoxicity if the ejection fraction falls by more than 10% on sequential scans.

d. It is possible to differentiate alcoholic from viral cardiomyopathy by gated blood pool imaging.

e. It is possible to differentiate ischaemic cardiomyopathy from dilated idiopathic cardiomyopathy with gated blood pool imaging.

A. 7.

a.   F   Patients with coronary artery disease typically show a fall or no increase in LVEF with exercise. Normal subjects show an increase in LV ejection fraction of 5% or more. Normal subjects over 60 may not show an increase in LVEF with exercise however.

b.   T   Any cardiac disease may affect ejection fraction. Coronary artery disease is usually of a more focal distribution whereas idiopathic cardiomyopathies cause diffuse involvement usually.

c.   T   This is a common indication for cardiac gated blood pool scans. A significant fall indicates that treatment should be stopped or irreversible cardiotoxicity may ensue.

d.   F   see b)

e.   T   see b)

Radionuclide ventriculography

Q. 8.

a. Radionuclide ventriculography is a more accurate and reproducible method for measuring ejection fraction than echocardiography.

b. Assumptions for the calculation of ejection fraction are greater for echocardiography than they are for radionuclide ventriculography.

c. In severe left ventricular dysfunction the volume of injected radiopharmaceutical is reduced to avoid overload.

d. Exercise ventriculography is not possible because there is too much motion of the patient.

e. It is not possible to measure right ventricular ejection fraction using gated equilibrium techniques.

A. 8.

a.   T   Echocardiography is more operator dependent and relies on a number of assumptions of ventricular geo-

b.   T   metry for calculating ejection fraction. These calculations are less accurate in badly impaired left ventricles.

c.   F   Unlike contrast ventriculography the injected volumes are tiny, typically less than 1 ml.

d.   F   This technique can be carried out using a bicycle ergometer in a semi-supine position. Straps can be used to minimise movement.

e.   F   This can be estimated but is less accurate than for the left ventricle. The main problem is overlap of activity in the right atrium and pulmonary artery and so first pass techniques may be better.

First pass radionuclide angiography

Q. 9.

a. It is possible to detect R to L cardiac shunts with this technique.

b. It is possible to detect L to R cardiac shunts with this technique.

c. As large a dilution of radiopharmaceutical as possible should be used in this technique.

d. It is an accurate technique to quantify cardiac shunting which coexists with coarctation of the aorta.

e. It is often not possible to accurately quantitate cardiac L to R shunts in the presence of tricuspid regurgitation.

A. 9.

a.   T   When frames are displayed in cine mode early LV and aortic filling can be seen. In addition there may be slow clearing of the lung due to the bi-directional nature of these shunts.

b.   T   Refilling of the RV and lungs without further clearance is seen. Shunt size can be quantified by measuring the pulmonary to systemic ratio of blood flow.

c.   F   A short, sharp bolus is required and the radio-pharmaceutical is given into the right antecubital fossa in less than 0.5 ml with a rapid flush with the arm abducted. If a ROI is drawn over the SVC this should give a bolus curve which ideally has a base of less than 3 seconds.

d.   F   Collateral arterial pulmonary supply may cause false recirculation peaks overestimating the size of L to R shunts.

e.   T   This will tend to split the delivery of the sharp bolus making quantitation very difficult.

Myocardial Infarct scanning

Q.10.

a. A myocardial infarction may be seen on an MDP bone scan.

b. ^{99m}Tc labelled pyrophosphate imaging may detect myocardial infarction before cardiac enzyme changes.

c. Rib fracture may give false positive results with pyrophosphate scanning.

d. Positive antimyosin monoclonal antibody scanning is specific for myocardial infarction.

e. Rejection of heart transplants can be detected with antimyosin scanning.

A.10.

a.   T   There is an influx of calcium into infarcted tissue. Pyrophosphate forms a complexes with calcium in damaged myocardial tissue and hence is able to localise in sites of ischaemic myocardial damage. MDP and pyrophosphate have similar chemical structures and MDP can also be seen to localise in infarcted tissue. Pyrophosphate has been used as a bone scanning agent in the past.

b.   F   Maximum sensitivity for detection of infarction is between 3 and 10 days although positive scans can be seen at 24 hours.

c.   T   see a) SPECT may help in this situation.

d.   F   Myosin is an intracellular myocyte protein which is only exposed to the extracellular environment during
e.   T   irreversible injury. This can then be detected by bonding with a monoclonal antibody directed against myosin. Acute myocarditis and heart transplant rejection will also cause a positive scan.

Chapter 7
Tumour Imaging

Gallium 67 citrate

Q. 1.

a. Gallium is rapidly bound to ferritin following injection.

b. Gallium is taken up into about 50% of lymphomas.

c. Benign processes do not usually accumulate Gallium.

d. In a patient who is breast feeding, uptake into the breasts usually indicates mastitis.

e. Visualisation of the kidneys before 24 hours usually indicates infection or inflammation.

A. 1.

a.   F   It rapidly binds to transferrin and images reflect the distribution of this protein i.e. reticuloendothelial system, liver etc.

b.   F   Sensitivities of greater than 90% have been reported. *Eur J Nucl Med*, 1990; 16:755

c.   F   TB, sarcoidosis and other infections and inflammations will accumulate Gallium. The mechanism of uptake is thought to be multifactorial.

d.   F   Breast uptake is commonly seen during lactation partly due to binding to lactoferrin. Breast feeding should be stopped indefinitely following a Gallium scan.

e.   F   The kidneys may normally be seen up to 24 hours but after this the likelihood of pathology increases. Imaging does not usually start until 48 or 72 hours, however.

Gallium 67 citrate

Q. 2.

a. Gallium is a useful agent for assessing inflammatory bowel disease.

b. Gallium is useful for distinguishing sarcoidosis from tuberculosis in the chest.

c. It is not possible to use SPECT for Gallium imaging due to the low count rates achieved.

d. A liver colloid scan is almost always required if investigating possible hepatic metastases with Gallium.

e. Gallium is particularly sensitive for necrotic tumours.

A. 2.

a.   F   There is normally visualisation of the large bowel with Gallium and so this limits its usefulness in the abdomen. Laxatives can be given to reduce bowel visualisation and sequential scans can be useful to confirm movement of gallium around the bowel in normal circumstances.

b.   F   There is high uptake into both of these diseases. The pattern of uptake may be of help however, outside the chest. Lacrimal and salivary gland uptake is very suggestive of sarcoidosis.

c.   F   A method for Gallium SPECT has been described using higher doses with SPECT to improve count statistics. *Ann Intern Med*, 1982; 66:694

d.   T   There is normal non specific uptake of Gallium into the liver making it more difficult to detect Gallium avid lesions. A cold lesion on a liver colloid scan which shows apparently normal Gallium accumulation is suggestive of tumour or abscess.

e.   F   Gallium uptake depends on tissue perfusion, increased permeability of tumour capillaries and delay in lymphatic new vessel growth. Necrotic, non perfused tumours will therefore not accumulate Gallium. *J Nucl Med*, 1986; 27:1215

MIBG

Q. 3.

a. MIBG is an analogue of cortisol.

b. ^{123}I MIBG imaging is the most sensitive method for detecting adrenal cortical adenomas.

c. ^{123}I MIBG imaging is less sensitive than bone scanning in detecting bone metastases in children with neuroblastoma.

d. ^{123}I MIBG imaging is more sensitive than CT in detecting extra adrenal metastases from malignant phaeochromocytomas.

e. ^{123}I MIBG imaging has a sensitivity of about 85% in detecting phaeochromocytomas.

A. 3.

a.   F   It is a noradrenaline analogue and this accounts for its uptake into catecholamine storage vesicles.

b.   F   It is used to detect adrenal medullary tumours e.g. phaeochromocytoma.

c.   F   MIBG is especially good in the bone extremeties where the distinction between metastatic disease and normal epiphyseal uptake may be difficult.

d.   T   Although CT sensitivity approaches 100% for 2 cm adrenal tumours, MIBG imaging is more sensitive for extra-adrenal tumours.

e.   T   In the clinical context of suspected phaeochromocytoma, specificity approaches 100%. *Clinical Nuclear Medicine,* Ch. 11

MIBG imaging is commonly used in the investigation of

Q. 4.

a.   carcinoid tumours

b.   glomus tumours

c.   small cell carcinoma of the bronchus

d.   paragangliomas

e.   nasopharyngeal tumours

A. 4.

a.   T

b.   T

c.   F

d.   T

e.   F

A wide range of neuroendocrine tumours with APUD and intracellular storage granules exist which take up MIBG. These include carcinoids, medullary carcinoma of the thyroid, paragangliomas, neuroendocrine granule containing Schwannomas, glomus tumours, Merkel cell tumours, bronchial carcinomas and neuroblastomas as well as phaeochromocytomas. The technique is not commonly used in bronchial tumours however.

Somatostatin analogues

Q. 5.

a. Octreotide has a shorter biological half life than somatostatin.

b. Somatostatin receptors are expressed on tumours other than those of neuroendocrine origin.

c. There are at least 3 types of naturally occurring somatostatin receptor.

d. Octreotide can be labelled with ^{99m}Tc.

e. Cold octreotide treatment should be stopped prior to labelled octreotide imaging.

A. 5.

a. F The biological half life of somatostatin is too short for imaging purposes and so the analogue octreotide is used which is much longer acting.

b. T In addition to neuroendocrine tumours somatostatin receptors have been found to be expressed on CNS, breast, lung and lymphomatous tumours.

c. T Type 1 — stomach and jejunum, type 2 — brain, kidney and pancreatic islets, type 3 — pancreatic islets.

d. F Only ^{111}In and ^{123}I as yet.

e. T This is usually the case as there is theoretical competition for binding sites between cold and labelled octreotide.

Labelled somatostatin analogues

Q. 6.

a. Can be used to investigate pituitary tumours.

b. Have a higher sensitivity for detection of carcinoid tumours than MIBG.

c. Can be used to investigate small cell carcinoma of the bronchus.

d. Nearly 100% of insulinomas may be identified with octreotide scintigraphy.

e. May prove useful in the evaluation of sarcoidosis.

A. 6.

a. T Between 75% to 100% of functioning and non functioning pituitary tumours may have somatostatin receptors. It has been found particularly useful in predicting which growth hormone secreting tumours will respond to cold octreotide treatment.

b. T Octreotide has a sensitivity in excess of 80% and so is better for tumour detection. As yet octreotide has not been labelled with a β emitting radionuclide and so radionuclide therapy still depends on ^{131}I MIBG.

c. T Approximately 80% of oat cell carcinomas of the bronchus exhibit somatostatin receptors and this technique may prove to be a useful staging and follow up procedure.

d. F Unlike gastrinomas and glucagonomas which show very high sensitivity only about 60% of insulinomas may be detected. This may be due to receptor subclasses present on this tumour.

e. T In one series 100% (23/23) of patients showed uptake of octreotide into sarcoid granulomata. *Eur J Nucl Med*, 1993; 20:716

Monoclonal antibodies (MAbs)

Q. 7.

a. Optimal uptake of radiolabelled MAbs occurs in large tumours in elderly patients.

b. Antibody fragments result in increased tumour detectability compared with whole antibody.

c. ^{111}In is considered the best radionuclide for labelling MAbs when hepatic metastases are being investigated.

d. SPECT may increase detection of tumours in MAb imaging.

e. MAb imaging techniques are particularly suitable for regular and long term follow up of tumours.

A. 7.

a.   F   Elderly patients are more likely to have multiple organ failures resulting in prolonged whole body retention and hence reduced tissue to background ratio. Large tumours are often partly necrotic and relative uptake is reduced in comparison to small tumours.

b.   T   This is probably due to increased clearance of fragments, so enhancing tissue to background ratios.

c.   F ^{111}In labelled MAbs tend to have a relatively high liver uptake and so tumours may appear less conspicuous.

d.   T   Low tissue to background ratios are a problem in MAb imaging and SPECT allows the separation of tumour from overlying non tumour activity.

e.   F   The MAbs are made from a mouse myeloma cell line and the development of human antimouse antibodies (HAMA) develops frequently on subsequent injections. HAMA result in altered kinetics with increased liver uptake and reduced tumour visualisation. Although adverse reactions have been reported on second or subsequent injections of a MAb they are relatively rare and are usually mild when they do occur. *Semin Nucl Med*, 1995; 25:144–164

Monoclonal antibodies

Q. 8.

a. MAb imaging has shown best results in detection of metastases from carcinoma of the breast.

b. Sensitivity and specificity of MAb imaging techniques are generally less than 50%.

c. The use of MAbs directed against CEA in colonic tumours is not worthwhile if circulating CEA levels are not raised.

d. Analysing the kinetics of areas of activity with respect to time increases the specificity of MAb imaging.

e. In the investigation of malignant melanoma with MAbs there is a poor detection of lesions of less than 2 cm.

A. 8.

a.   F   Most experience exists for gastrointestinal tumours, carcinoma of the ovary and melanoma.

b.   F   The average sensitivity and specificity from a number of gastrointestinal MAb studies were 79% and 85% respectively.

c.   F   Although sensitivity is reduced compared to when circulating CEA levels are high, it was found to be 63% in one study.

d.   T   Activity in tumours was found to increase over 22 hours whereas areas in which activity reduced corresponded to vascular structures.

e.   T   70% of the lesions that are missed are less than 2 cm.
Semin Nucl Med, 1995; 25:144–164

Miscellaneous tumor imaging

Q. 9.

a. ^{99m}Tc V DMSA is a useful radiopharmaceutical for staging squamous cell carcinomas of the head and neck.

b. ^{99m}Tc V DMSA is a useful radiopharmaceutical for staging of medullary thyroid carcinoma.

c. Labelled red blood cell imaging of the liver with SPECT is a highly sensitive method for diagnosing haemangiomas of less than 1 cm.

d. Liver haemangiomas appear hot in the first minute of imaging with labelled red blood cells because they are so vascular.

e. Primary brain tumours usually show a hot spot on ^{99m}Tc HMPAO imaging.

A. 9.

a.   F   Pentavalent DMSA is prepared as renal DMSA but in an alkaline solution. It has been shown to have in-

b.   T   creased uptake in a number of tumours. Although up-take can be seen in squamous cell carcinomas of the head and neck, imaging with this agent has been shown to be not superior to clinical examination. (*Nucl Med Commun*, 1989; 10:239). Sensitivities approaching 90% have been reported with medullary thyroid carci-noma however and this agent is probably the imaging agent of choice at present in patients with suspected recurrence. (*J Nucl Med*, 1988; 29:33–38)

c.   F   Above 1 cm red blood cell SPECT compares favourably with MRI but sensitivities fall off below this size due to the inferior spatial resolution of nuclear medicine tech-niques. (*J Nucl Med*, 1993; 34:375–380).

d.   F   The characteristic appearance is similar to that of dy-namic contrast enhanced CT. A photon deficient area is seen in the early stages which gradually becomes as in-tense as the normal liver. On delayed images it will ap-pear as a hot spot due to the increase in blood pool in comparison to the liver.

e.   F   In contrast to blood-brain-barrier imaging HMPAO (cerebral perfusion) usually shows reduced uptake in comparison to normal cortex. (*Nucl Med Commun*, 1986; 7:274)

Miscellaneous tumour imaging

Q.10.

a. Anterior mediastinal uptake of Gallium in children following chemotherapy almost invariably signifies recurrent disease in lymphoma.

b. Gallium imaging should take place immediately after chemotherapy.

c. Thallium may be used to differentiate tumour from reactive gliosis in primary brain tumours.

d. Adrenal carcinomas show increased uptake of seleno-cholesterol.

e. The thyroid gland is usually well seen in 131-I MIBG imaging.

A.10.

a.   F   Chemotherapy may cause thymic rebound which shows uptake of Gallium.

b.   F   False negative results may occur. This is thought to be due to increased iron binding to transferrin, displacing Gallium.

c.   T   Positive uptake will occur in recurrent tumour. (*J Nucl Med*, 1991; 32:962)

d.   F   The carcinoma is not usually sufficiently differentiated and does not take up enough tracer to be imaged. The contralateral adrenal cortex is suppressed. Absent uptake of tracer in the adrenal areas results.

e.   F   The thyroid gland would be seen if uptake was not routinely blocked. It is anticipated that there will be a small percentage of free iodine with MIBG and the thyroid is therefore routinely blocked with substances such as potassium iodate to reduce uptake into this radiosensitive gland.

Chapter 8

PET Imaging

CNS

Q. 1.

a. ^{18}FDG is an analogue of glucose labelled with ^{18}F.

b. FDG enters and takes part in biochemical pathways in exactly the same way as glucose.

c. Malignant tumours show as hot spots with FDG PET because they generally have a higher glycolytic rate than normal tissues.

d. Brain tumours commonly show as relative cold spots.

e. The degree of uptake of FDG into a primary brain tumour correlates well with the histological grade of tumour.

A. 1.

a. T   Fluorodeoxyglucose behaves in a similar fashion to glucose but only takes part in the first step of Krebs

b. F   cycle. It then remains trapped in cells in amounts proportional to the glycolytic rate. ^{11}C methionine is also taken up in increased amounts in malignant tissue, the exact mechanism being uncertain.

c. T   As one would intuitively expect. PET is probably the most reliable way to differentiate viable tumour from post treatment gliosis. Gliosis shows low grade or absent FDG metabolism (or ^{11}C methionine uptake).

d. T   Normal brain cortex has one of the highest metabolic rates for glucose and therefore low grade tumours may appear relatively cold.

e. T   This obviously has prognostic implications. FDG PET may also therefore detect dedifferentiation of tumours.

In epilepsy

Q. 2.

a. FDG PET most commonly shows an area of increased metabolism at the site of an epileptogenic focus.

b. FDG PET is more sensitive than ^{99m}Tc HMPAO SPECT in identifying epileptogenic foci in temporal lobe epilepsy interictally.

c. FDG PET is the method of choice rather than ^{99m}Tc HMPAO SPECT in identifying epileptogenic foci in temporal lobe epilepsy intraictally.

d. If MRI is abnormal in TLE there is no further information to be gained by performing FDG PET in addition.

e. Increased benzodiazepine receptors are usually seen at epileptogenic foci.

A. 2.

a. F Most scans are performed interictally at which time a hypometabolic focus is usually seen. FDG PET is more
b. T sensitive than HMPAO blood flow SPECT in locating foci, at least in part due the better resolution. It is logis-
c. F tically very difficult to perform ictal PET and so this is not the method of choice. Ictal SPECT is less difficult logistically and is regarded as one of the best non invasive methods of lateralisation of TLE prior to surgery. Ictal scans characteristically show increased blood flow or metabolism at the focus.

d. T *J Neurol*, 1987; 234:377–384

e. F Less uptake of ^{11}C flumazenil at epileptogenic foci has been described in keeping with the hypothesis that there is reduced inhibition at the ictus. (*Neurology*, 1995; 45:934–941)

Oncology

Q. 3.

a. Lymphomas characteristically show marked uptake of ^{11}C methionine but poor or absent uptake of ^{18}FDG.

b. FDG PET has a similar accuracy to CT in the preoperative staging of carcinoma of the bronchus.

c. FDG PET has a similar diagnostic accuracy to mammography in the differentiation of benign from malignant lesions.

d. Melanomas show avid uptake of FDG.

e. In the early post radiotherapy assessment of primary malignant brain tumours, increased uptake of FDG nearly always indicates residual disease.

A. 3.

a.   F   Both radiopharmaceuticals show avid uptake into lymphomas. (*J Nucl Med*, 1991; 32:1211–1218)

b.   F   FDG PET is more sensitive. One third of patients deemed operable by CT criteria may have unsuspected metastases which can be identified with PET. In one study 18% of patients had management altered to a non surgical regime. (*Lancet*, 1994; 344:1265–1266)

c.   F   PET appears to be very sensitive and specific with figures approaching 100%. (*Radiology*, 1993; 187:743–750)

d.   T   PET appears to be good for staging and follow up. (*Radiology*, 1995; 195:705–709)

e.   F   Following radiotherapy there may be an inflammatory reaction. Macrophages may show quite high uptake of FDG and the inflammatory reaction may give the false impression of residual tumour unless the scan is appropriately timed. ^{11}C methionine is a better agent for early post treatment evaluation. (*J Nucl Med*, 1995; 36:484–492)

The following are true

Q. 4.

a. It is only possible to perform cardiac PET studies in close proximity to a cyclotron because of the short half lives of PET radiotracers.

b. Pharmacological stress is best avoided in cardiac PET studies because of interactions between the stress agent and radiotracer.

c. Ischaemic myocardium shows poor uptake of FDG.

d. PET may identify hibernating myocardium.

e. Diabetic patients have particularly good quality FDG scans because of their high circulating blood sugar.

A. 4.

a.   F   If there is an on site cyclotron then it is possible to use $^{13}NH_3$ for blood flow studies but rubidium-82 (a potassium analogue, similar to thallium) can be obtained from a generator system.

b.   F   PET cardiac scans rely mostly on pharmacological stress (dipyridamole, adenosine, dobutamine) as exercise is difficult to perform in the scanner.

c.   F   Myocardium usually utilises glucose and fatty acids but switches predominantly to glucose when ischaemic. Ischaemic tissue may therefore show preserved or even increased accumulation of FDG.

d.   T   PET is probably the best non invasive technique to identify hibernating myocardium i.e. myocardium with diminished blood flow and poor wall motion which is not distinguishable from infarcted tissue by most imaging methods but which may regain function on revascularisation. If FDG uptake is preserved in an area of diminished or apparently absent blood flow, the myocardium can be said to be viable. Regions showing this pattern are able to function again after revascularisation in contrast to a completed infarct which shows absent perfusion and metabolism.

e.   F   With high blood sugar and low insulin levels there is very poor uptake of FDG resulting in poor quality scans. Insulin may be given to "drive" FDG into the myocardium and improve scan quality.

Chapter 9
Miscellaneous

Concerning the biodistribution of ^{99m}Tc-HMPAO

Q. 1.

a. ^{99m}Tc-HMPAO crosses the blood-brain barrier.

b. Regional uptake of HMPAO is proportional to regional cerebral blood flow to the same area.

c. Distribution of HMPAO in the brain is independent of brain maturation.

d. Diffuse lung uptake of HMPAO is seen only in people with a history of smoking.

e. Focal cerebral uptake is seen in herpes simples encephalitis.

A. 1.

a.   T ^{99m}Tc-HMPAO is one of a newer group of lipophilic tracers which cross the blood brain barrier and localise and remain in normal brain tissue. The older BBB imaging agents (DTPA, glucoheptonate, pertechnetate) are non-lipophilic and only cross the BBB if damaged.

b.   T   Approximately 60% (the lipophilic portion) of the injected dose is available for extraction by the brain cells; they receive HMPAO via the arterial supply and extract approximately 85–90% of the HMPAO delivered to them at first pass. Therefore regional uptake of HMPAO is proportional to the cerebral blood flow. (*Clinical Nuclear Medicine*, Ch. 7)

c.   F   In SPECT studies performed on infants of increasing ages, immature neonates (younger than 40 weeks gestation) show prominent uptake in the thalamus and basal ganglia and relatively little cortical uptake; with increasing age parieto-occipital cortical activity appears and frontal cortical activity is dominant at 6 months.

d.   T   Diffuse pulmonary uptake of HMPAO is only seen in the lungs of current or ex-smokers and correlates strongly with smoking history. Focal uptake may be seen in squamous cell and adenocarcinoma of the lung.

e.   T   Focal areas of cerebral uptake is seen in brain tumours (primary or metastatic), focal areas of infection (such as herpes simplex encephalitis and opportunistic infections in immunocompromised patients) and focal areas of functional disturbance (complex partial seizures, schizophrenia). (*Semin Nucl Med*, 1994; 24:180–182)

Brain SPECT

Q. 2.

a. The distribution of ^{99m}Tc HMPAO reflects regional glucose metabolism.

b. ^{99m}Tc HMPAO has to be used within 30 minutes of being prepared.

c. It is helpful to create images in the axis of the temporal lobes when investigating temporal lobe epilepsy.

d. Bright lights or loud sounds at the time of injection may alter the distribution of ^{99m}Tc HMPAO.

e. It is possible to accurately assess the size of the lateral ventricles with brain blood flow tracers.

A. 2.

a. F HMPAO is a lipophilic agent which readily enters brain cells but then changes to a more hydrophilic substance which cannot diffuse out again. It is therefore distributed according to regional cerebral blood flow (rCBF) and because of this has been termed a "chemical microsphere".

b. T It is relatively unstable *in vitro*.

c. T Scans are acquired digitally and can therefore be reconstructed in any plane. It is often helpful when investigating temporal lobe epilepsy to reconstruct additional slices in the longtitudinal axis of the temporal lobes.

d. T Anything which alters regional cerebral blood flow will alter the distribution of tracer. A standardised environment is recommended and it has been found that injections with eyes open and the ears unplugged with low ambient noise and light produces the least variability. (*Radiologic Clinics of North America*, 1993; 31:881–907)

e. F There is poor uptake of these tracers into the white matter and the ventricular system and it is not possible to differentiate the boundary between them.

Concerning dementia

Q. 3.

a. Increased accumulation of cerebral blood flow tracers is seen in the frontal lobes in Picks disease.

b. Abnormalities in Alzheimer's disease are often bilateral and predominantly affect the temporal and parietal lobes.

c. AIDS dementia complex usually shows no abnormalities on brain SPECT imaging.

d. Typical blood flow changes are seen in the basal ganglia in asymptomatic patients with Huntington's chorea.

e. A characteristic pattern of reduced rCBF is seen in idiopathic Parkinsons's disease.

A. 3.

a.   F   Symmetrical reduction is the typical pattern.

b.   T   Changes may be asymmetrical however. Typically, there is sparing of the sensorimotor and visual cortices, subcortical regions and cerebellum.

c.   F   They are nearly always abnormal and usually demonstrate focal or multiple areas of decreased uptake affecting predominantly the frontoparietal regions. The scan is sensitive but not specific. Improvements can be seen following treatment with AZT.

d.   T   The typical pattern is of decreased uptake in the caudate nuclei corresponding to atrophy at this site. The appearances are strongly suggestive of Huntington's chorea particularly when a family history is present. Hypoperfusion of the basal ganglia may also be seen in Wilson's disease and Fahr's disease, however.

e.   F   No characteristic basal ganglia changes are noted. (*Radiologic Clinics of North America*, 1993; 31:881–907)

Concerning lymphatic and lymph node scanning

Q. 4.

a. Non-visualisation of a lymph node group means that it is diseased.

b. Both hot and cold spots may be abnormal.

c. One advantage over lymphangiography is that the internal iliac nodes are usually seen.

d. Approximately a third of studies for nodal involvement will be inconclusive.

e. In Milroy's disease, colloid pools in the feet.

A. 4.

a.   F   Lymph nodes may not be visualised either because they are absent (normal anatomical variation) or because they are diseased and it is usually not possible to say which is the case.

b.   T   Both hot and cold spots can be abnormal because when lymph nodes are infiltrated, the phagocytes can be stimulated (and therefore take up more colloid), depressed or replaced.

c.   F   Neither lymphoscintigraphy or lymphangiography demonstrate the internal iliac nodes or provide information about the immediate lymphatic drainage from the lower urinary or reproductive tracts.

d.   T   Approximately 30% of studies will give an inconclusive result, but lymphangiography and CT also have their own disadvantages. Infection and radiotherapy will interfere with image interpretation.

e.   T   In Milroy's disease (congenital absence of lymphatics) the colloid pools in the feet without progressing further. (*Clinical Nuclear Medicine*, Ch. 21)

Concerning lymphoscintigraphy and tumour surgery

Q. 5.

a. It may be used pre-operatively in patients prior to tumour and nodal dissection to define lymphatic pathways.

b. Sentinal nodes may be identified by intra-operative lymphoscintigraphy.

c. In head and neck melanomas there is a high agreement between drainage sites which would have been predicted by the conventional approach and those demonstrated by scintigraphy.

d. The ultrasound and mammographic findings are used to identify the most appropriate injection site.

e. In breast cancer approximately 1/3 of tumours show unexpected drainage across the centre of the breast.

A. 5.

a.   T   Pre-operative lymphoscintigrams are being used increasingly in some centres to assess lymphatic drainage pathways and nodal involvement which would not have been predicted from a conventional approach.

b.   T   Intra-operative scintigraphy has been used to identify sentinal nodes to be dissected, but this needs to be performed under standardised conditions to be validated.

c.   F   Head and neck melanomas have unpredictable drainage pathways with high disagreement (64–73%) between predicted and demonstrated nodal drainage sites — especially important as surgery in this area is likely to be very disfiguring. For truncal melanomas the agreement is slightly greater (44–54%).

d.   T

e.   T   In a recent study, 32% of inner or outer quadrant lesions showed unexpected drainage across the centre of the breast to axillary or internal mammary nodes. (*J Nucl Med*, 1995; 10:1780–1783)

Concerning testicular scanning

Q. 6.

a. After the injection of radionuclide in testicular torsion an area of reduced or absent uptake is seen on the affected side.

b. In epidydimo-orchitis an area of reduced or absent uptake is seen throughout the scrotum.

c. A ring of activity surrounding a photon deficient area may be seen in torsion.

d. A hydrocele may cause a false negative result when scanning for torsion.

e. Teratomas may show specific uptake of tracer.

A. 6.

a.   T   Following testicular torsion, typically, scrotal scintigraphy shows reduced or absent activity following
b.   F   intravenous injection of ^{99m}Tc pertechnetate on dynamic vascular phases and on blood pool, equilibrium
c.   T   images. As the time since torsion increases, a hyper-
aemic rim of increased activity may be seen. In con-
d.   F   trast, epidydimo-orchitis shows a pattern of diffusely
increased blood pool activity on the affected side. The
technique carries sensitivities of more than 95%.
Specificity is reduced by other conditions causing an
intrascrotal photon deficient area such as hydrocele or
haematoma.

e.   F   This is not an indication for scrotal scintigraphy.
(*Radiology*, 1977; 125:739–752, *Semin Nucl Med*, 1990;
20:159–188)

Miscellaneous: sialoscintigraphy and lymphoscintigraphy

Q. 7.

a. ^{99m}Tc pertechnetate is the agent of choice for studying salivary gland function.

b. Parotid, submandibular and sublingual salivary gland function may be assessed.

c. Lymphoscintigraphy can show increased passage of tracer towards the groin in venous oedema.

d. Lymphoscintigraphy allows the differentiation of limb swelling due to venous and lymphoedema.

e. The sensitivity for detecting lymph nodes with metastatic disease is nearly the same as for contrast lymphography.

A. 7.

a.   T ^{99m}Tc pertechnetate is available directly from a generator. It is readily taken up into salivary glands (as well

b.   F   as thyroid, stomach, choroid plexus, kidneys etc). The sublingual glands are too small to resolve but the parotid and submandibular glands are easily identified. By drawing regions of interest around the four glands, time activity curves can be produced. This allows relative function to be compared and allows assessment of gland excretion following a sialogogue. This functional information may complement the largely anatomical information from contrast sialography.

c.   T   Increased lymphatic drainage may result to compensate.

d.   T ^{99m}Tc nanocolloid is injected into a web space of a limb subcutaneously on both sides and is subsequently taken up into the lymphatics. By scanning dynamically it is possible to follow the passage of tracer through the lymphatics. By quantitating uptake into the groin nodes it is possible to differentiate lymphoedema from venous oedema and normals. (*Clin Nucl Med*, 1993; 18:646–654)

e.   F   In general this is not true as the resolution of the technique is not good enough to identify nodes which are infiltrated as in lymphography. However in one situation, the assessment of the internal mammary chain, isotope lymphography has proven better than MRI or CT in detecting diseased nodes. By injecting at the xiphisternum diseased nodes may be identified by reduced uptake, contributing to the staging of breast cancer. (*Clin Nucl Med*, 1992; 17:482–484)

Miscellaneous: Dacroscintigraphy and breast imaging

Q. 8.

a. In dacroscintigraphy failure of passage of radiotracer through the lacrimal duct indicates mechanical obstruction.

b. If lacrimal ducts are patent on syringing, there is no need to carry out dacroscintigraphy.

c. Epiphora may result in rapid disappearance of tracer from the eyelids.

d. ^{99m}Tc sestamibi breast imaging may reliably differentiate benign from malignant breast lesions.

e. ^{99m}Tc sestamibi breast imaging detects axillary metastases with a sensitivity as good as that for the primary lesion.

A. 8.

a.   F   Functional as well as mechanical causes will show absent or delayed passage of tracer through the naso-

b.   F   lacrimal duct when instilled into the lower lid. Syringing of the ducts only confirms that they are not completely obstructed. It does not exclude partial mechanical or functional obstruction.

c.   T   Tear production may be so great that tracer may spill onto the cheeks rather than passing down the nasolacrimal ducts giving a false impression of rapid clearance.

d.   T   One study reports a sensitivity, specificity and accuracy of 84,100 and 87% respectively in 38 patients (32 malignant, 6 benign). (*Eur J Nucl Med*, 1994; 21:432–436)

e.   F   Another larger study showed uptake in only 8 out of 14 involved axillary nodes. (*Nucl Med Commun*, 1994; 15:604–612)

Appendix: The PIOPED Study

To date the largest prospective trial to assess the role of V/Q scanning in pulmonary thromboembolism is the PIOPED study (JAMA 1990; 263:2753–59). Pulmonary angiography was carried out in 933 patients and was used as the gold standard. Interpretation criteria were modified from those of Biello in order to give every patient a diagnostic category. Large defects were defined as >75% of a lung segment; moderate defects 25–75% and small defects <25%.

High Probability
1. >2 large defects of perfusion without corresponding V or CXR abnormality.
2. 1 large segmental plus >2 moderate defects without corresponding V or CXR abnormality.
3. >4 moderate defects without corresponding V or CXR abnormality.

Indeterminate Probability
1. 1 moderate to <2 large defects without corresponding V or CXR abnormality.
2. Corresponding V/Q defects and CXR abnormality in lower zone.
3. Corresponding V/Q defects and small pleural effusion.
4. Single moderate matched defect with normal CXR.
5. Difficult to categorise as normal, low or high probability.

Low Probability
1. Multiple matched V/Q defects, regardless of size. CXR normal.
2. Corresponding V/Q defects and CXR abnormality in upper or lower zones.
3. Corresponding V/Q defects and large pleural effusion.
4. Any perfusion defect with substantially greater CXR abnormality.
5. Stripe sign.
6. Single or multiple small perfusion defects. CXR normal.
7. Non-segmental perfusion defects.

Normal
1. Normal perfusion scan.

   Inter-observer variability was low for high probability and normal or near normal scans (8% and 5% respectively). However, observers found greater difficulty in classifying scans as low or intermediate probability and agreed only 75% of the time. The addition of the clinical evaluation to the scan result improved the risk stratification of patients suspected of having PE.

Conclusions
1. Normal perfusion excludes clinically significant PE.
2. Low probability scans with low clinical probability of PE and no evidence of venous thrombosis do not require further study or anticoagulation.
3. Low probability scans with intermediate or high clinical likelihood of PE require venous studies of the lower limbs. If positive they should be treated.
4. Stable patients with an indeterminate scan and high clinical probability of PE may need venous studies or angiography.
5. Stable patients with a high probability scan and clinical probabilty for PE require treatment and no further tests to confirm the diagnosis.
6. Stable patients with a high probability scan and low or intermediate clinical probability of PE may require venous studies of the legs, and if these are normal, pulmonary angiography.

Bibliography

Radiology Review Manual: 2nd Edition, Wolfgang Danhert *Williams and Wilkins 1993*

Bone Scanning in Clinical Practice, I. Fogelman *Springer Verlag 1987*

Gamuts in Nuclear Medicine, Frederick L. Datz *Mosby Year Book 1995*

Clinical Nuclear Medicine: 2nd Edition, MN Maisey, KE Britton and DL Gilday. *Lippincott Raven Pub. 1991*

An Atlas of Clinical Nuclear Medicine: 2nd Edition, I. Fogelman, MN Maisey and SEM Clarke *Mosby Year Book 1994*

Nuclear Medicine in Clinical Diagnosis and Treatment: IP Murray and PJ Ell eds. *Churchill Livingstone 1995*

Printed in the United States
by Baker & Taylor Publisher Services